Chelation Can Cure

Chelation Can Cure

Dr. E. W. McDonagh, D.O.

Platinum Pen Publishers, Inc.

Platinum Pen Publishers, Inc.
Box 11127
4810 N.E. Vivion Road
Kansas City, Missouri 64119

First Printing 1983
Second Printing 1987
In the United States of America

Library of Congress Cataloging in Publication Data
McDonagh, E. W. (Edward W.), 1932-
    Chelation Can Cure.
    Bibliography: p.
    1. Ethylenediaminetetraacetic acid—Therapeutic use.
2. Chelation Therapy. I. Title.
RM666.E845M34   1983   615'.31   83-4107

ISBN 0-912815-00-0

To the women I live with,
who make my life worthwhile,
this book is affectionately dedicated:

Norma Jean
Jamie Sue
Jodi Ann

Many people helped to make this book possible. I am especially indebted to: Sara Stonner, Debbie Hoggatt, and Kelly Seute, for the daily aid they provided. Mr. Calvin Jones of Radio Shack, who spent many hours of his free time at my home helping me unsnarl the idiosyncrasies of my word processor used to write parts of this book, deserves special thanks.

I sincerely thank all of these fine people.

Table of Contents

v

FOREWORD

Mainstream medicine chooses not to recognize the great benefits of EDTA chelation.

To wait until deterioration is so great that the patient is forced to undergo drastic measures such as bypass surgery, or transplant surgery, is needlessly tragic. These cruel assaults are mostly unnecessary. No longer should treatment after the fact be tolerated by an enlightened public. The amputated leg or foot in many cases need not have been removed. Coronary artery bypass surgery can be eliminated in 80 to 90% of cases.

Heart disease, vascular occlusive disease, strokes, arthritis, senility, kidney disease, gangrene, diabetes and the complications of these dreadful afflictions have been successfully treated and reversed by doctors using a treatment method known as EDTA Chelation Therapy.

The results McDonagh Medical Center has been able to demonstrate with thousands of patients for more than twenty years have been duplicated time and time again in clinics scattered across this country.

This story screams for attention. EDTA Therapy can enable "untreatable" patients to return to health, to rise from their own ashes of deterioration.

1

The State of the Art in Mainstream Medicine

In September 1982, a study was published in the *Journal of the American Medical Association* that simply had to be embarassing to cardiologists and internal medicine specialists. It revealed that patients with heart disease treated with conventional drugs died earlier than patients with the same type of heart disease who took no drugs.

In the United States, treatment after the fact is the usual medical approach. Results are speculative because the amount of disease in the patient determines the percentage of improvement. The most talented doctor in the world cannot get favorable results in a severely compromised patient, one who has several diseased organ systems.

Surgeons must keep a certain batting average to maintain surgical privileges at the hospital. Hospitals want patients to survive surgery. They can't afford otherwise. Surgeons and most specialists therefore rigidly select the patients they accept for treatment. If a patient seems too big a risk, they will not accept the case.

What happens to the untreatable cases? The usual method is to place the patient on drugs to control pain and other symptoms. This, of course, does not get at the cause of the problem, and so the patient continues to slide. His life ebbs until he dies.

Imagine how you would feel if you discovered a fire in your living room tonight. When the fire department answers your call, the fire chief says, "It's too little for the men to fool with. Call us again when the flames are shooting through the roof."

Conventional medicine chooses this philosophy when it comes to treating chronic diseases. Patients have to be seriously ill to be treated, and by that time several of their systems have been compromised. This approach is responsible for the unchecked growth of circulatory disease, high blood pressure, heart attacks, strokes, diabetic complications and a host of other degenerative metabolic diseases. Yet this type of thinking is used by our government, hospital associations, medical associations and health insurers. It is one of the major reasons this country has such a poor record with degenerative diseases.

One method of treating cardiovascular disease is the rather late hospitalization of the patient in a special coronary care unit, where the needs of heart attack victims are catered to exclusively. Most of the 7,000 general hospitals in the U.S. have coronary care units (CCU). Specialized coronary care for heart attack victims can reduce in-hospital deaths by about 30%. That is, they can save three out of ten CCU admitted heart attack victims.

Another popular method of relieving the heart patient of his life-threatening coronary occlusive disease is bypass surgery. If a patient survives the initial attack and has been stabilized by the CCU, or if a patient has had diagnosis before a heart attack, this surgery is recommended by cardiologists and heart surgeons as the treatment of choice for his problem. More than 57,000 coronary artery bypass surgeries were performed in 1975, and by the end of 1983 the annual number had grown to 191,000.

A decade of scientific study has shown that except in certain well-defined situations, bypass surgery does not save lives or even prevent heart attacks.

The New England Journal of Medicine has reported several studies indicating that no more than 21% of the total bypass operations can be considered effective. More than 79% of these procedures make no helpful change in the lives of the hopeless patients who undergo this serious operation. A 1977 study by the Veterans Administration—and a duplicate study in 1978 by the National Institute of Health—detected no difference in the rates of survival for those who have bypass surgery and those who do not, unless the patient suffers from an obstruction of the left main coronary artery, a particularly severe form of heart disease.

Bypass surgery patients have a 2% risk of dying on the operating table. They have a 5% risk of heart attack during the operation. And they have a 5 to 10% chance of serious complications such as stroke. The operation does not cure anything and in many cases a second operation is required within ten years.

According to an *Atlantic Monthly* article, coronary bypass surgery consumes more of this country's medical dollars than any other procedure. It cost the American public $5 billion in 1983. The average cardiac surgeon's fee is between $4,500 and $5,000 per bypass operation. Five or six bypass operations a day are not unusual. Professional fees for cardiac catheterization, a basic test often done two or three times for each surgical patient, average $800 each.

Cardiac operations are the biggest revenue producers for hospitals. These institutions get $1,000 a day, plus extras for intensive care units, $5,000 to $8,000 for operating room fees, $1,100 lab fees, and they make many other charges. The total hospital bill will average $25,000 per patient. In some cases total charges can reach $100,000.

In the United States, we do bypass surgery twice as often as it is done in Canada and Australia, four times more than the rate in Western Europe. Is it any wonder the motives of cardiac surgeons, cardiologists and the hospitals are extremely suspect?

Bypass surgical results are not permanent. One reason is because the surgeon takes a piece of the saphenous vein from the patient's leg, and uses it to channel or jump around the occluded portion of the coronary artery. Veins, however, are not designed to carry blood under high pressure. Arteries are.

Unlike arteries, there are no heavy muscular walls in veins. When bypass surgery is completed, and the new vessel graft is forced to carry high pressure blood from the heart, deterioration begins. The elastic fibers and collagen fibers in the wall begin to stretch beyond their structural limits. When the intimal lining on the inside of the grafted vessel can stretch no more, small tears occur. Calcium, always present in the bloodstream, enters the vessel wall through these small intimal injuries.

Calcium is a divalent metal. Due to its two positive charges, electromagnetically it attracts fats and proteins from the blood to itself. A sticky sludge is formed at the site of the small injury in the vessel wall. Additional calcium infiltrates, and more fat and protein along with cellular debris, platelets and other material keep the vicious cycle cooking. The plaque so formed continues to bulge into the vessel interior, narrowing the space available for blood transport. Electromagnetic attraction enables the plaque to extend for some distance down the length of the vessel.

A kindergarten student can easily demonstrate the forces involved using a small magnet, a piece of paper and some iron filings. Once spread over the paper, iron filings will not move. If the child places the magnet under the paper, the iron filings will bunch and pile up over the area influenced by the magnet.

Ballooning of the vein graft by high pressure arterial blood is the culprit. Intimal tears enable divalent calcium to enter the wall and begin the atherosclerotic process. The question remains, should a vein designed to carry low pressure blood be used to carry high pressure blood in the first place? The smooth, slick surface of the normal intimal lining has been interrupted during the surgeons stitching of the ends of the new graft vessel. This area too, is a major site for the buildup of the atherosclerotic plaque. Commonly, it builds up at the sites where it was sewn in.

When this happens the patient again has his old problems

back: chest pain, shortness of breath, increasing fatigue, and so on. At this point he is usually advised to have bypass surgery again. This scenario is repeated until there is no more room for additional vessel grafts. Our hapless patient is now advised that nothing more can be done. He is referred to the internist or cardiologist for drug palliation. He continues rapid deterioration, loses more function, has more pain, and finally exits this life.

Another reason surgery doesn't live up to expectations is today's medical philosophy. Contemporary physicians choose to treat symptoms of disease, rather than causes. When the coronary artery becomes occluded inside, and the blood supply downstream to the heart muscle is sufficiently restricted pain results (though not always), function suffers, and the patient is in danger of myocardial infarction (heart attack). Something must be done. In some cases surgery is the emergency treatment. There is ample evidence, however, that the coronary artery bypass operation is grossly overutilized. Marsha Millman, in her book, *The Unkindest Cut,* presents facts that indicate this surgery actually contributes to worsening of the heart wall muscle.

The surgeon does not effectively aid more than a few inches of the occluding artery in any case. Mile after mile after mile of arteries, veins and capillary vessels continue to lose their ability to carry the blood in sufficient quantities due to the atherosclerotic process. Surgery can never hope to be an effective method for relieving the sludging and crusting inside blood vessels. It is stop-gap, Band-Aid treatment at best. It is doomed to failure.

To believe otherwise is foolish. It would be like the little ten fingered Dutch boy trying to stop twenty-five leaks in the dam. The battle to restore health has not even begun, let alone won, by a risky, expensive surgery.

On March 15, 1981, in San Francisco, the 30th Annual Scientific Session of the American College of Cardiology, began an organizational meeting. It lasted five days and was attended by 14,000 health care professionals. Nine thousand of them were cardiologists.

Emilio R. Giuliani, M.D., Professor of Medicine at Mayo Medical School, Rochester, Minnesota, was co-chairman of this meeting. Summing up the findings and conclusions of the numerous papers presented, Dr. Giuliani was quoted as saying:

"It is difficult to spot arteriosclerosis early. It presents no symptoms and develops slowly over a period of years. The condition usually goes undetected until it produces a heart attack or stroke. All too often, sudden death occurs before any sign of clogged arteries appears.

"Every patient, on becoming symptomatic, should first be treated with every medical means available. Only those patients who fail to respond to the maximum medical programs available should be considered for surgery. The great majority of patients with coronary artery disease are not candidates for saphenous vein bypass surgery.

"Present data suggest that only a small number of these patients benefit from bypass surgery. This includes patients with critical lesions involving the main coronary artery and patients with all three major artery involvement with critical diseases or lesions. Patients undergoing surgery must have adequate runoff vessels, as well as adequate ventricular function. Further, continued medical management following surgery is essential. This includes treatment of hypertension, obesity, diabetes; avoiding nicotine and caffeine and excessive use of sugar, salt and fats.

"In brief, for all those patients who have clinical coronary disease—even those for whom surgery plays a role—long-term broad medical [holistic] treatment is the most important aspect of management. The only effective treatment, however, is prevention."

Another way doctors approach the difficult problem of cardiovascular disease is by prescribing drugs. When a patient is suffering from atherosclerosis and segments of his arterial system are plugging up, dilator drugs—and there are many different varieties—are used.

An article in *Wall Street Journal*, Friday, August 6, 1982 stated that Minnesota Mining and Manufacturing Company would be marketing a new heart drug, Tambocor. The drug was undergoing clinical trials in the United States and would be submitted to the Food and Drug Administration for approval by early 1983. The diversified maker of adhesives estimated the cardiovascular therapy market in the U.S. at an annual $1.6 billion.

With a market this size, and growing, it is unlikely that the United States will attempt to deemphasize the drug treatment idea. Drugs serve to dilate (expand) the normal segments of a vessel, but unfortunately they are ineffective in plugged areas. They cannot act on the inside wall of the artery if it is insulated by an occluding ring of fats, cellular debris, calcium, etc. This approach is useless as a treatment for atherosclerosis.

Other drugs aimed at reducing cholesterol and fat buildup inside the artery are generally expensive, ineffective and doomed to failure unless the fat intake of the patient is reduced drastically. Do physicians emphasize this to patients strongly enough?

Drugs are used more effectively in the control of high blood pressure. The key word here is control. Drugs do not eliminate the cause of the elevation in blood pressure, or of cholesterol. When they are effective, drugs treat the symptoms or end results, leaving the initiating cause untouched.

The state of the art in mainstream medicine should not be what it is. It need not be that way. You, the reader, must *arm* yourself with the knowledge necessary to demand EDTA Chelation Therapy as an alternative to surgery.

This book will provide knowledge of what chelation treatment with EDTA is, and how it helps patients back to health. It will present convincing case histories of how persons with certain chronic diseases were able to have their condition reversed. These case histories come from my personal experience at the McDonagh Medical Center. I, personally know the reporting to be factual.

2
What is Chelation

The term *chelation* (kee-LAY-shun) comes from the Greek word *chele* for claw. A simple technical explanation of chelation is that it involves the incorporation of a metal into a heterocyclic ring structure by a chelating agent. The chelating agent attracts the metal to its molecular structure with an electromagnetic charge. When the metal joins the molecular structure of the chelating agent, the result is a closed ring. After this process takes place, the metal is said to be "chelated." The metal is now part of the new structure, trapped inside the ring, and has a new identity. It loses all its former toxic properties and is, in effect, a captive of the chelating agent.

The chemical principle of chelation is used in many industrial processes, such as water softening. It is the mechanisms of action of some commonly used detergents. Soluble chelates are formed with such bases as calcium and magnesium and are much more effective than soaps. These new products do not leave the usual ring of scum in the bathtub, nor do they harm clothes, as soap will do.

The action of many successfully used drugs is based upon chelation activities. Chelating agents developed during the last twenty or thirty years, initially used exclusively to rid the body of toxic heavy metals, recently have been shown to possess great effectiveness for the treatment of such diverse conditions as contamination by radio-isotopes (radiation), the prophyrias, digitalis induced cardiac arrhythmias, scleroderma, metastic calcium deposits in various body tissues (e.g., nephrocalcinosis, kidney stones, prostatic calcinosis, calcific bursitis, tenosynovitis), and the atherosclerotic plaques which result in occlusive vascular disease with subsequent tissue ischemia and metabolic failure.

Among the chelating agents now in use for various therapeutic purposes, one of the most effective for the removal of calcium from living tissues is the disodium salt of ethylene diamine tetraacetic acid, also known as disodium edetate, and edethamil disodium.

The innumerable enzyme systems in every living organism from bacteria to man are formed through chelation. Enzymatic activities of all living cells are carried on through chelation exchanges of ions, such as in the metabolic pathways for the transport of iron absorbed from food in the gastrointestinal tract up to its destination in the molecules of hemoglobin, or as in the migration of ingested zinc to form part of the molecules of insulin.

Vitamins C and E are natural chelating agents. The amino acids, the body's building blocks, are also chelators. These natural nutrients are not strong enough when taken in the usual dietary amounts, to clean the narrowed blood vessels. Their function is mainly to enhance or maintain normal circulation. Once circulation is blocked, however, stronger chelating agents are needed. Nutrients from your daily food intake are handled by a chelation process. They are dissolved, absorbed and bound to proteins so they can be transported unhampered to their final destination.

A solid like your child's lollypop is changed from solid to liquid by his constant licking, and though still present in another form, the candy is transported harmlessly to the stomach, eventually to be absorbed into the blood and finally across the cell membranes into the cells as sugar. Without this process the lollypop could not enter the cells.

Plants and animals depend upon chelation to obtain and use metals. Chlorophyll, the green part of plants, is a chelate of magnesium. Hemoglobin, peroxidase, cytochrome C and catalase are chelates of iron. Many successful drugs used to treat disease are dependent upon chelation processes for their effectiveness. More detailed information is contained in an excellent book by Bruce W. Halstead, M.D., *The Scientific Basis of Chelation Therapy.* I recommend this book for the technically oriented reader.

Ethylene diamine tetraacetic acid (called EDTA for the sake of brevity) is a non-toxic amino acid that was synthesized in Germany in 1931. It was designed to treat severely lead poisoned patients. Prior to its development, there was little that could be done for these unfortunate people. They died because of the tremendous toxic effect of lead on the brain, nervous system and other major organs.

Chemists in the food processing industry are quite familiar with chelation chemistry and EDTA. The research literature contains more than 3,000 reference papers concerning EDTA. EDTA is used as a preservative in countless foodstuffs, canned, bottled, and dry packed.

The chemistry of blood banking is another source of EDTA information. The substance is used in the performance of many blood tests. Banked blood has small amounts of EDTA added to prevent blood cells from breaking down.

EDTA is known to be a calcium blocking agent, a potent coronary vasodilator. In other words, EDTA can bind or chelate calcium as well as other minerals in the body. It will remove calcium particles deposited in arterial wall plaques and atheromas. In addition, EDTA blocks the slow calcium currents in the arterial wall, resulting in arterial vasodilation.

To review precisely what chelation is, consider the following: The electromagnetic attraction of fats and proteins for divalent calcium that has wandered through the injuries in blood vessel walls, is the same process that enables EDTA to remove calcium and fat from the plaque that occludes the vessel. A study of over six hundred human aortas has demonstrated alterations in the elastic tissue with accumulations of calcium prior to the deposition of fat and cholesterol. (Blumenthal, 1944).

Calcium has two positive charges which are called valences. Hence, calcium is divalent. Calcium is strongly attracted electromagnetically by the open-ended, molecular structure of EDTA that is circulating in the blood during the chelation treatment. This results in the calcium ion being incorporated into the EDTA molecular structure, forming a closed ring. When this process takes place, the metal is said to be *chelated* and EDTA is termed the *chelating agent.*

When calcium (or other divalent metals such as lead, mercury, cadmium, aluminum, etc.) is chelated by EDTA, the original electromagentic attraction is lost, and the fatty debris is dissolved by circulating blood and metabolized.

The calcium-EDTA molecule, now inactive and non-toxic, is carried by the blood until it passes through the kidneys. It then is removed from the body via the urine.

The solid sticky plaque goes into solution and is harmlessly removed. By this unique mechanism, dangerous solids are converted to a liquid, then transported away to be eliminated. This is a natural, normal phenomenon of body chemistry.

Norman E. Clarke, Sr., M.D., a cardiologist at Providence Hospital in Detroit, was the first American to discover the many beneficial effects of EDTA chelation. When he treated battery factory workers for lead poisoning, they reported relief of their symptons of chest pain (angina), arthritis, intermittent claudication (severe leg pain due to plugged arteries in the legs), as well as their symptoms of lead poisoning.

Dr. Clarke, now in his eighties and very active in practice and on the lecture circuit, is recognized as a chelation pioneer in the Soviet Union. The Russians use chelation therapy as the second most common treatment for arteriosclerotic artery disease.

It is also the preferred method of treatment in Czechoslovakia. EDTA chelation is administered with great success for blood vessel disease, stroke, senility, diabetes, kidney diseases, and other degenerative diseases in Germany, Switzerland, Mexico and Canada, to name just a few countries.

The 1972 Czechoslovakian article, *Chelates in the Treatment of Occlusive Atherosclerosis,* concluded that EDTA was the treatment of choice for vascular disease producing claudication (pain in legs when walking).

The pharmacology of EDTA and its toxicity were reviewed in 1959 by Muller, Brynsting and Winklemann. They found the drug to be 69 to 92% effective for the removal of metastatic calcium from various body tissues, and free from significant side effects when properly administered. They also observed that EDTA is rapidly eliminated intact as a chelate ring—without any metabolic breakdown—in urinary and fecal excretions.

The potential uses of chelation in cardiovascular disease were reviewed by Kitchell, Meltzer and Seven when they attempted to explain the mode of action as chiefly involving modifications of metabolic functions, not only of calcium and zinc, but perhaps of many other trace metals. They observed that calcareous lesions of the heart and aortic valves, as well as the intimal calcinosis (innermost lining of the blood vessel), could dissolve during EDTA infusion therapy.

In March of 1963, *Medical World News* published an interview which quoted Dr. Kitchell as saying, "Peripheral vascular occlusive disease of the smaller blood vessels shows remarkable changes following treatment with EDTA. Candidates for below-the-knee amputation have lost their gangrene. One ended up walking seven miles when he could not walk a block before."

An associate of Dr. Kitchell, Dr. Meltzer, reported: "Eleven out of twelve patients with vascular disease secondary to diabetes have improved, and considering the absence of any · valuable method for treating diabetic vascular disease, chelation therapy must assume great importance." He also hoped the treatment would avoid many of the amputations currently required due to gangrene.

The effectiveness of EDTA for the removal of calcium from intimal atheromatous plaques was demonstrated by Bolick and Blankenhorn in a study which also showed that coronary atheromata may contain as much or more calcium per unit of weight as do advanced aortic or iliac arterial lesions.

Recent reviews of therapeutics pay a great deal of attention to EDTA. Chemically, calcium is a metal and is the most abundant and accessible bivalent cation in the body, taking part in the production of many types of degenerative disorders that Virchow called "metastatic calcium deposits."

These disorders are the subject of a more recent study by Selye, 1960, in the development of his theory of calciphylaxis. His experiments seem to indicate that one of the basic phenomena leading to aging and other damaging changes in living tissues is the metastatic deposition of calcium. It frequently becomes highly desirable to remove some calcium from the body, and it has been amply demonstrated that EDTA can perform this task safely and efficiently.

Our experience at McDonagh Medical Center leaves no doubt that properly administered, EDTA produces remarkably beneficial effects on the human body. Every cell benefits. Results are seen first in the blood vessels, notably the arteries. EDTA, dripped slowly into a vein, has the advantage over surgery of being able to reach all sites of vascular occlusion in the body at the same time.

Abnormal calcium is removed, and the occluded vessels are reopened. This effect is produced only upon metastatic calcium (calcium found in areas where it should not be), and not upon normal tissue calcium, as shown consistently by the lack of development of osteoporosis or of increased dental caries. Increased x-ray bone density is observed in cases of osteoporosis after they have been treated with EDTA. Lamar has described the reduction in visible aortic calcification with simultaneous apparent recalcification of previously osteoporotic vertebral bones.

This process may go on for months and explain the frequently described phenomena of continued clinical improvement after chelation has ceased, such as improved joint function, as arthritic joint deposits are decreased.

Some critics have complained that treatment with EDTA is not "permanent."

These uninformed experts would know, if they had any experience with the treatment, that the results are probably more permanent than any other vascular treatment utilized in this country today.

Serum cholesterol concentration is determined before and during therapy. In all cases, abnormally high cholesterol is normalized.

Pulse volume recordings of the arteries before and after treatment prove easily the improvement in the inside diameter of the vessel tested. These results correlate with the increased pulsations of the arteries in all areas of the body, and with clinical and metabolic evidence of improvement. Once the occluding slag and sludge is removed from the inside walls of the arteries they can carry blood efficiently once more, and elasticity returns. In other words, ischemic atherosclerosis is reversed.

Parenteral administration of EDTA frequently improves conduction mechanisms in first degree, second degree, and advanced heart block. It abolishes ectopic ventricular contractions and terminates ventricular tachycardia. It increases the rate of idioventricular pacemakers in complete heart block.

On January 8, 1970, the Food and Drug Administration referred to calcium or disodium EDTA as follows: "The drug is possibly effective in occlusive vascular disorders and the treatment of pathologic conditions to which calcium tissue deposits or hypercalcemia may contribute other than those listed above."

At that time our Federal Drug Administration recognized and approved the use of EDTA chelation treatment in circulation diseases. Since then the agency has changed its position, not because there is scientific evidence that EDTA is unsafe, but for political reasons alone.

Between 1970 and 1982 more than three million doses for EDTA have been given safely, and with excellent results. In 1983, it was estimated that more patients had EDTA chelation treatment than had coronary bypass surgery. For more details the reader is referred to three excellent books on the subject by Harper, Walker, and McDonagh.

Tissues, organs and cells downstream of the formerly plugged artery can now obtain the nutrients and oxygen once denied. These cells once dormant, or partially dor- mant, can now revive and carry on their normal metabolic chemistry. Toxins and waste products that have not been properly removed due to inadequate circulation are eliminated as the perfusion normalizes.

3

How Does Chelation Therapy Work?

During the early 1960s, when I was learning the EDTA chelation treatment method, I hospitalized all patients for thirty days of EDTA treatments. They were given a month's leave from the hospital, then re-admitted for an additional thirty days of treatment. All patients received a liter (about one quart) of EDTA solution dripped into the vein for a minimum of four hours. Many of the most severely ill patients had the treatment time extended to five to six hours.

The patients were confined to bed, except for bathroom usage.

Medically, they suffered from advanced heart disease, diabetes, stroke, gangrene, high blood pressure and circulatory failure of various organs. For the two years that I treated patients with EDTA in this manner, not one had a venous thrombosis.

Some patients required surgery. The majority were able to obtain excellent recovery without surgical intervention. Most of these patients were over sixty years of age.

It is common medical practice in some circles for certain severely ill patients to be screened out and tactfully sent home, rather than offered treatment. The reasons for rejecting them as patients are not pleasant to relate. Many doctors and hospitals need to show a high success rate. To accept such patients who will probably die in spite of treatment, or who will likely not survive a proposed operation, would be to build a bad mortality record. So to avoid a high death rate statistic, the procedures are performed only on patients who are stronger, who are more likely to get well.

During the years that I have been privileged to observe patients before, during and after chelation treatment, I have found rigid selection of patients (rejection of those whose disease was too avanced) was not necessary. Those patients who expected to get little if any treatment results from conventional medical treatment could get good to excellent results from EDTA chelation.

With only minor exceptions, patients with advanced chronic disese are suitable candidates for chelation treatment. Those excepted would be the unmanageable patient, the comatose patient, or the patient who could not function in an office or outpatient setting.

I am continuously amazed at the ability of the most severely ill human body to regain normal function.

I believe the "point of no return" is able to be stretched quite far for the severely ill chronic disease patient. A chronic disease is one with any loss of function, or illness, that has not been completely eliminated by medical treatment. It is a disease state that will continue to deteriorate in spite of drug control. Examples include arthritis, vascular disease causing high blood pressure or circulation loss, diabetes, heart disease, senility, etc.

EDTA chelation, monitored prescribed exercise programs, vitamin and mineral supplementation, dietary changes and the elimination of health hazards such as tobacco, caffeine, alcohol, excessive fat, sugar and salt, all add their part to the healing process.

On the other hand, the 5% of patients evaluated and judged to be at or past the "point of no return" are treated in this manner also. In addition, they are placed on conventional treatment that would be given by any hospital or doctor, and might include drug therapy. The combined treatment approach is very fruitful. There is a synergism when using the two together. One plus one equals five—that is, the overall treatment result is greater than the sum of the individual effects.

EDTA chelation treatment can help those very advanced chronic diseased patients and in the majority of cases bring the patient back to normal function. The treatment can clean up the blood vessels and organs in even the most severely ill patients, and many times the patient can then be successfully treated with the usual conventional treatment. Another common medical practice in this country is that of treating patients only when they exhibit symptoms of chronic illness. The rule seems to be, "If it's not broke, don't fix it." Which is fine, as long as it's someone else's health that needs to be "broken." How much better would it be if we could spend more resources and attention on keeping people well, rather than concentrating on trying to make people better after they are sick.

A growing number of physicians, including myself, feel that we should concentrate our attention on staying well. Holistic medicine prefers to help people quit smoking, lower cholesterol in their diets, reduce hypertension and exercise more. If we spent more effort on prevention, we would not have to spend so much on exotic surgical techniques.

If health planners would only rethink their philosophy of approach—unencumbered and uninhibited by present problems—I believe progress could be made in the health care for the United States citizen. We should concentrate on health improvement and maintenance. We should not wait until the citizen has a disease before he is eligible for aid from the system.

By teaching the people the early signs and symptoms of chronic disease, how to live, what to eat, how to exercise, what to avoid, health and longevity can be favorably improved. Incentives to keep healthy need to be devised.

Screening procedures for vascular disease, heart disease, and most other chronic degenerative disease can now be performed in the doctor's office, if he cares enough, in the earliest possible detection of these terrible sappers of life and function. They can be done easily, and noninvasively.

No longer is it necessary to go to a hospital for expensive invasive testing. In such procedures an artery is pierced and dye injected, then many x-rays are taken to determine the inside diameter of the blood vessels. These tests are painful, require anesthesia and/or sedation, and impose considerable risk. We have seen many patients who have suffered an embolism in a distant organ such as a kidney or lung. During these procedures one elderly gentleman had this test because of coronary artery occlusive disease. His chest pain was getting worse in spite of drug therapy. During the angiographic procedure, small pieces of debris were apparently knocked loose from inside a blood vessel and this man didn't awaken for three months. He had suffered a stroke on the operating table. He came to our clinic with slurred speech, weakness in one arm and leg, and loss of mental function and memory. He was successfully treated with EDTA therapy.

Treatment with EDTA has many advantages that conventional medicine can never offer. This treatment can...

1. Treat several areas of illness in the body at the same time.

2. Be combined with drug, antibiotic or other therapy to treat the disease conditions. The patient makes a faster response, and can then be weaned from drug therapy. Chelation and supplementation can complete the recovery.

3. Eliminate the need for hospitalization for most chronically ill patients.

4. Greatly reduce the costs to patients (or their insurers) for drugs.

5. Keep wellness (health) intact longer, once it has been attained.

6. Greatly increase the effectiveness in the treatment of heart disease, stroke, diabetes, gangrene, retinitis, macular degeneration, kidney disease, and many other difficult medical conditions. (Medicine today is less effective than it could be in these areas.)

7. Salvage millions of minds and bodies of working people who have potentially killing or incapacitating disease smoldering in their systems. These are citizens supporting the economy. Should they drop out of the system prematurely, the remaining taxpayers must support them.

8. Withstand the test of time. For the more than twenty years that I have been personally involved with EDTA treatment, results such as those presented in this book have been obtained consistently. Many other physicians provide confirmation.

Patients who have not reached a crisis in their health can be diagnosed early, before serious impairment occurs. Once discovered the natural approach with EDTA will enable the body to reverse the disease process and will return the patient to optimum health. This healthy patient will reach a much higher state of wellness than is possible under the current mode of drugs/surgery therapy. It will last longer, too.

Unfortunately, the hospital is the last place one could expect to have health maintenance performed for him. Health insurers will not permit the physician to test outside the area of the chief complaint. This is an attempt to keep the size of claims to a minimum and to move patients out of the hospital quickly. The idea is laudable, but the methods used are laughable.

The way to keep medical claims to a minimum, is to keep hospital admission to a minimum. This is done by keeping people healthy, not by waiting until they are falling apart.

Any piece of machinery has a maintenance schedule. Your new car has definite time schedules for oil, lubrication and other preventive maintenance procedures. Without such care, the machine will not last the length of the guarantee. Is the body that much different?

A person seeking to find a way to enhance longevity and optimal health must go to a clinic that has experience in this manner of human medical care. More physicians will offer this type of practice if the public will demand it.

An editorial by Harry Schwartz in the *Wall Street Journal*, April 21, 1980, entitled, *Medical Costs and the Drug In-*

dustry, states in part:

"For years now Americans have been exhorted to realize there is no infinite source of resources to give everybody all the medical care he or she might want. We shall have to decide who may live and who must die in making medico-economic decisions, we have been told, and even some Congressmen have been heard criticizing the federal program that pays for kidney dialysis and transplants because it benefits all comers regardless of age, occupation, social usefulness or what have you."

Scary Orwellian rhetoric, isn't it?

It would seem federal thinking is indicating that modern medicine for all its chrome-plated gimmickry and rocketing costs cannot get the job done. Are only those rich persons who can afford the cost, or only those who meet certain government requirements to be given treatment? Must we now accede to a monumental cop-out and let people die?

This is why it is important for you to know about EDTA treatment. It is safe. It has been amply documented, and this process of documentation continues. It works. It is very inexpensive.

It will prevent the tragic loss of you or your loved ones if you take advantage of your new knowledge. It will prevent the vegetative half-life of the chronically ill and disabled.

4

Why Isn't Chelation Therapy Adopted By Everyone

Nasty politics and dirty laundry is not a subject for this book, yet both are historical facts. In this book I shall endeavor to tell the things I am personally acquainted with, and cite our own scientific research. We have published twenty papers attesting to the great benefits of this natural approach to degenerative disease. Many of the details in those papers will appear throughout this text.

People and organizations that would lose business if chelation therapy became a common office procedure by physicians have done their very best to keep this treatment from the public.

Surgeons, cardiologists, and internists would naturally feel somewhat threatened if 90% of the chronic illness could be reversed in the early stages.

Drug companies want to continue bringing to market dozens of drugs that are only temporary help at best. Drugs that control the symptoms are more profitable than a treatment that would eliminate the need for drug use. Sometimes drugs slow the progress of the disease a bit, but the disease marches on nevertheless.

In present-day chemotherapeutics, calcium antagonists are receiving a big play, with the introduction of several *new* drugs that do on a small scale things that EDTA has been doing for decades. Drug companies can patent the newer entities. EDTA is too old to patent. Once patented, millions are spent ballyhooing the *new* drug to doctors. Profits swell.

Hospitals want to keep their beds full so they can justify their existence. They can't afford to run in the red. They have large overhead expenses. At this writing there is a surplus of hospital beds in Kansas City, Missouri, and many of the larger hospitals are advertising for patients in a variety of ways. It's a safe bet they don't want to recommend a treatment that will keep patients away from the hospital.

Health insurers also are under the gun, in this era of high prices. They continue to diminish the benefits of their premium paying policy holders by denying payment for more and more conditions. They have been heavily pressured by powerful hospital organizations, by medical organizations such as the surgeons' groups, the internists' organizations, the cardiologists' societies, and other medical establishments.

What it boils down to is, modern medicine cannot deliver the goods to the paying patient. As a result the cost cutters have begun to deny patients the coverage for which they have been paying and doctors are not permitted to do thorough workups and treatment. The insurers and the hospitals want you in and out in as short a time as possible. The claims are smaller this way, and the hospitals can realize more income, for the first day or two are the most profitable for any hospital due to the testing done at that time.

Government regulating agencies take advice from panels of physicians. Human prejudice is easy to get, but very hard to lose. It dies with great difficulty. When physicians are prejudiced against chelation treatment, you can imagine the advice they give the government. The government (no small insurer of Medicare patients in this country) is only too eager to find a reason to deny payment for this treatment with the hope of reducing benefits for patients over sixty-five.

Because agencies fail to bring home the bacon to tax paying consumers as promised when politicians were looking for votes, medical treatment will continue to miss the mark. Costs will continue to skyrocket as treatment results plummet. The weeping, gnashing of teeth, and buck passing has already begun.

In his book, *Chelation Therapy*, Doctor Morton Walker states:

"There are powerful forces at work in our country to suppress this important medical discovery. For many different reasons united only by a combination of ignorance, arrogance, and greed—the medical establishment, the political establishment, drug companies, and the health insurance industry have combined to deny this treatment to you and your loved ones."

The medical establishment is worried. It seems to be running scared. Why else would its practitioners threaten people who have had coronary artery bypass surgery with loss of medical attention if we were allowed to inform them about EDTA treatment? It appears the establishment would do anything necessary to save its ego, integrity, veracity and, of course, its incomes.

Present-day medical planners must be enlightened and made knowledgeable of this treatment method. Physicians comprising the planning committees that advise governing and regulating authorities should be aware of EDTA chelation benefits.

Social Security is in financial trouble. Social programs cost more than strapped budgets can tolerate. Pensions from the armed forces and private companies are rapidly becoming eroded, riddled, shot through and moth-eaten by the voracious appetite of inflation.

A recent front page article with a Washington dateline in the *Arizona Republic* newspaper underlines a problem the federal government is having with costs of medical care:

"A Senate House committee agreed...to a hefty cut in the tax deduction for medical expenses and to elimination of the flat $150 write-off for health insurance premiums.

"The action may mean higher taxes for many of the 18 million couples and individuals who claim deductions for insurance and other medical and dental expenses. The changes would cost those taxpayers $3.8 billion over the next three years."

There is no real method operating to keep people alive and functional as long as possible, and at the same time help the bureaucrats out of the present medical cost-benefit dilemma.

On the other hand, if EDTA chelation treatment were administered early in the development of chronic disease, there would be huge savings in the medical budget. The grim reaper's harvest could be slashed drastically. People living longer, advancing in their jobs, professions and businesses would greatly stem the loss of brainpower and earning power necessary to develop new markets, new technology and new answers to other problems.

The economy needs more consumers and more taxpayers. When people are lost to tax rolls as a result of chronic disease, those who remain pay more than their share of taxes. They cut down on other items because they have less disposable income. Manufacturers cut back, store keepers suffer, and we have the negative economic situation we see in the national economy today. On the other hand, keeping more people alive, happy, working, buying and paying taxes, puts the economy on a positive footing, and makes expansion the dominant psychology. This can be accomplished simply by keeping our population healthy and free from diseases and degeneration.

Because the fruits of chelation therapy are not sufficiently recognized by medical planners, it becomes the duty of others to carry the fight forward, win widespread acceptance for it, then gather the healthful harvest.

Important, significant changes usually are brought about as a result of public pressure. If you want your family, your friends, or yourself to be able to live long without suffering the ravages of chronic disease, you must take up the banner and fight. Inform your friends about EDTA treatment. Inform your physicians that you desire the treatment as an alternative to the usual drug or surgery recommendation. Inform politicians and legislators on all levels of your findings and desires. Ask those who oppose chelation to cite either scientific evidence or studies on human beings that prove chelation does not work. There are none.

Are steps being taken to keep the sickness care systems healthy, instead of the populace? If all doctors could use the treatment, would too many hospitals lose too many patients? Would drug companies suffer losses of sales? Are the regulating agencies compromising our health system to commerce?

You must decide these questions. Stranger things have developed in government. The tobacco subsidy is an example. We support the price the farmer gets for his tobacco crop, and we have assistance programs to erradicate the pests and other dangers to the plants. All this while the Surgeon General of the United States warns the people that tobacco is detrimental to the health of users.

We have a national policy that discourages the use of addicting drugs by our citizens, and have strong enforcement agencies with a mission of detection and prosecution of drug sellers. Nevertheless, alcohol, the most widely used and abused drug in this nation, is looked upon with equanimity. People who promote alcohol, and those who sell it are considered to be in legitimate businesses, even though alcohol related automobile deaths "normally" number nearly 30,000 yearly.

There are many more examples of this schizophrenic dicotomy in our national priorities. You, the tax paying, voting citizens must let our office-holding politicians know what type of health care program you want.

If you are satisfied with the present method of dispensing medical care only after you are significantly sick, do nothing. If you believe, as we do, that the time to intercede is at the point of earliest detection, tell the legislators, and tell them frequently. They will listen to the voice of people who employ them.

Organize letter writing campaigns among your family and friends, church groups, unions, etc. Remember, every elected official from the president to the local dog catcher works for you, and is paid with your hard earned dollars.

So, with a few generalized statements concerning the medical establishment off my chest, let me answer a few specific comments that come from opponents of chelation therapy.

The *Harvard Medical School Health Letter* states, "There is no credible evidence that chelation therapy works as claimed." The rest of this book will be devoted—disease by disease—to a history of our experiences relating how chelation therapy has saved lives and made thousands of people feel better.

To the scientific community, these histories are anecdotal, not scientific studies. To do scientific studies on the level these opponents would require would cost $10 to $30 million. We have already shown that drug companies, hospitals and specialized physicians are not going to jeopardize their profits by sponsoring such studies.

You should know that standard medical treatments, including coronary bypass surgery, have been introduced without vigorous testing. Doctors want to help their patients. If a procedure appears to help save lives, why not use coronary bypass surgery? Both methods appear to save the lives of patients. In the section on heart disease, I will have more to say about the effectiveness of coronary bypass surgeries in light of current research.

Another objection to chelation therapy is made because no "double blind" studies have been done. This procedure divides patients into two groups: one group, let's call it group A, gets the medication being evaluated, and the other, group B, gets a placebo that appears identical to the active drug, but in fact is without substance.

Those administering the study do not know which patients are getting the placebo or the medication due to a coding procedure. Finally the patients are tested and results are evaluated.

The test is repeated, with group A now getting placebo medication, and group B getting the active medicine. When the code is broken after completion of the study, those patients getting the active medication are identified. Theoretically, this should prove or disprove that improvements were caused by the test medicine.

There are several criticisms of this procedure, and scientists are divided in their opinion about double blind testing methods. Two common objections to the system are as follows:

1. In a private practice, it would be unethical to charge for placebo treatment. If a charge is not made, the test would not be valid. Those paying the fee would know they were getting the active medication. The others would have obvious psychological input into the test, thereby invalidating it.

2. There have been no double blind studies of the coronary artery bypass surgery, possibly the most overutilized surgical procedure in America, yet it is accepted as worthwhile by medical and government authorities, and approved for payment by insurance companies. Apparently double blind studies are not truly necessary.

Our clinic has published papers demonstrating that renal function is actually improved by chelation therapy. We have also published papers establishing proper dosages, determined by years of experience and observation in working with these procedures. When used in proper dosages, there are absolutely no dangerous side effects from using EDTA.

There are very few chemotherapy drugs in use today for which such a claim can be made. All drugs must be administered with care. We have not had a death at McDonagh Medical Center for more than fifteen years that could be attributed to EDTA chelation therapy.

Some critics claim that EDTA is toxic to the kidneys. The charge is made that treatment results are not "permanent," as if traditional approaches to heart and artery diseases were ever permament.

Those who would have you believe chelation is dangerous or ineffective should be totally ignored, unless they have had personal experience in administering this form of medical treatment. If they have never treated a patient with EDTA, or even seen a patient before and after chelation therapy, their advice is hearsay. Any lawyer or judge in this country can tell you quickly how much heresay statements are worth.

If you think suppression of EDTA treatment is not intentional, quick reading of *The Great Medical Monopoly Wars,* by P.J. Lisa, will clear the air. This book documents the unethical and immoral propaganda that a small but powerful and well financed segment of the medical community is using to keep from the public knowledge that might promote health.

Medical establishment bureaucrats have often suppressed freedom of speech in an effort to thwart the dissemination of chelation information.

Dr. Charles J. Rudolph, Ph.D., D.O., my partner in McDonagh Medical Center, Inc., is highly qualified in biochemistry, having earned his Ph.D. in that field at Oklahoma State University. He was graduated with honors. He is medical director for mineral analysis laboratories in Texas and New Mexico. He has written and published several papers in the field of nutrition and trace mineral supplementation. He was invited to speak at the Missouri Association of Osteopathic Physicians and Surgeons (MAOPS) meeting held at the Hyatt Regency Hotel, Kansas City, Missouri, in the spring of 1981, by Mr. Edward Borman, secretary of that organization. Several hundred physicians were in attendance at the lectures. Before Dr. Rudolph began his lecture, the meeting room cleared, except for three courageous physicans. They had heard him speak before knowing the high quality of his presentations and decided to risk the wrath of their colleagues who were boycotting his lecture.

Dr. James Critchlow owns a small pharmaceutical company in Cooper City, Florida. This company offers high quality vitamin and mineral preparations, glandular products, enzymes, etc. He had supported MAOPS for several years by purchasing display booth space at their meetings. His company also sells EDTA and that product was on display. As the meeting got underway, several doctors told him that MAOPS did not like EDTA treatment and the *word* was out to boycott his booth. When he asked what they knew about the treatment, no one had even rudimentary knowledge of its benefits or mechanism of action. "Then why are you slamming something you know nothing about?" said Jim. "We were told to," was the reply. Dr. Critchlow, after learning of Dr. Rudolph's plight on the lecture platform, informed us of his experience.

I was to speak to a meeting of interested citizens at Clinton, Missouri, on March 10, 1982. Mrs. Doris Bowen, assistant administrator of our clinic, made several calls and a trip to Clinton arranging for the lecture. On the night of the talk, three of us made the fifty mile drive to Clinton. The building had been nicely set up, with microphone in place, lectern, chairs, everything ready. One small problem. No one showed up for the speech in spite of advanced notice and promotion. We had expected fifty or more. The lady custodian of the building was very pleasant to us. She eventually told us how the Clinton residents were coerced into participating in this boycott, giving up their rights—in my opinion—to hear about EDTA treatment. It seems one of the members of the city council was opposed to EDTA chelation. He had served on the peer review committee of Blue Cross-Blue Shield, an organization that does not recognize chelation treatment. The city fathers let it be known, according to this lady, that no one was to attend this free lecture.

The Mended Hearts, an organization formed by four patients who had survived heart surgery in 1951, was incorporated under the laws of Massachusetts in 1955. The pamphlet, *Heart to Heart From the Mended Hearts, Inc.,* states in the paragraph titled "Aims of the Mended Hearts, Inc.": "To give help and encourage others who are faced with or have had heart surgery." "To assist in research programs seeking the causes and cures of heart disease." The pamphlet further states Mended Hearts are "keenly interested in the advance of medical knowledge that means renewed lives for so many people...[and] are endorsed by the American Heart

Association, its affiliates, and by numerous institutions and agencies throughout the United States. Many surgeons now recognize the value of the unusual service that only Mended Hearts can offer their patients."

Mended Hearts have over one-thousand chapters in this country. The Kansas City chapter, number eighty-six, has one hundred members. Mended Hearts, I feel, are being used as a propaganda agency for the American Heart Association, those stalwart surgeons who, it would seem, love to do bypass operations. The AHA provides regular lecturers to Mended Hearts meetings. I have attended a meeting during which an AHA member spoke.

From volume six, issue number five of the *Heartland Newsletter,* printed under the letterhead, "The Mended Hearts, Inc., Heart of America, Chapter number eighty-six, serving the Kansas City Metropolitan Area," dated October 7, 1981, comes a hint of the possible propaganda exploitation to which members have been lulled. From the program announcement: "The doors will be opened at 6:30 p.m. Training for candidates, and study for accredited visitors will begin at 6:45 p.m."

Before a member can volunteer service to give a reassuring talk to a hospitalized patient about to have coronary bypass surgery, he must be accredited, that is, he is told what to say to "reassure" the patient. Could the canned speech really be aimed at keeping the patient from changing his mind? The paragraph under "Program" continued: "Dr. E. W. McDonagh, D.O., Director and Founder of McDonagh Medical Center, Gladstone, Missouri. Dr. McDonagh will discuss "Chelation Therapy, an Alternate for Arteriosclerosis." We believe you will find this a most informative and enjoyable program and it is hoped that you will invite a friend to share the evening with you. Continued discussions whether on a question and answer basis or another friendly chit-chat will be an impromptu or as-you-care-to basis."

The night before I was to speak, I received a call from the president of chapter eighty-six. She said she was withdrawing my invitation to speak due to the "large amount of misinformation concerning chelation therapy."

"Have you heard about EDTA chelation treatment?" I asked. "No, I haven't." "Then how can you judge the information until you do?" I asked.

I asked her to permit the members and their guests to judge the information after I presented our data slides and after I spoke, not before. She refused.

An internal memo of McDonagh Medical Center, signed by the administrator and business manager, Mr. William D. Johnson, dated October 13, 1981, is reproduced totally. It capsulizes the truth:

"At 8:50 a.m. I spoke with Mr. Ruebelmann, Vice President of the Mended Hearts Association and was informed that they had not denied Dr. McDonagh the right to speak, but were told in no uncertain terms by the American Heart Association and the American Medical Association that if they were, in fact, to allow Dr. McDonagh to appear before the Mended Hearts group they would forego their right to enter any hospital in the Kansas City area and that the American Heart Association and the American Medical Association would withdraw their support of the group. Dr. McDonagh was scheduled to speak to the Mended Hearts group on October 13, 1981 at 7:30 p.m."

Such petty attempts at censorship should be beneath the dignity of such organizations. I find it hard to believe that these societies have jettisoned ideals that for many decades have shown them to be dedicated leaders in the fight against disease. It appears that present-day leaders are stooping to gutter levels. The medical associations mentioned are not hopelessly flawed, I prefer to believe, but they have people problems.

Our clinic continues to add new patients daily as the word continues to spread, patient to patient, about the reversal of disease brought about by chelation therapy. Those few "forbidden" speaking engagements are usually rescheduled at another time, on our own territory, and they are very well received.

5
Chelation Therapy
And Cardiovascular Disease

Cardiovascular disease is usually without symptoms in the majority of patients until it becomes well established. In more than 25% of patients, coronary occlusive disease has no warning or pain before sudden death strikes. Early examination by a physician using sufficiently sophisticated testing equipment is necessary to show abnormal changes in the arteries, veins, or heart early enough to intercede and reverse the disease. All of us should consider the known risk factors of cardiovascular disease. High blood pressure, cigarette smoking, plasma low density lipoprotein cholesterol, stress and hardness of drinking water can be changed.

Cigarette smoking has clearly been shown to be a potent risk factor for coronary, cerebral (brain) and peripheral blood vessel disease. Sudden death, heart attack, angina, claudication and stroke incidence and prevalence can be related to the number of cigarettes one smokes per day. The greater the number, the higher the risk. If you smoke, stop being foolishly influenced by other smokers and by advertising media.

Stop smoking, even though it might be difficult. I empathize with those who have become addicted to tobacco. Twenty years ago, before I quit, I was smoking three packs of cigarettes per day.

The four chambered hollow muscular organ that occupies the center of your chest and pumps a continuous flow of blood throughout the circulatory system is your heart. Each day the heart beats 100,000 times and pumps 4,300 gallons of blood. This is the equivalent of seventy-eight 55-gallon barrels of blood, a remarkable work load for an organ about the size of your fist.

The heart is divided into a right and left side. Each side has an atrium, a chamber in which blood collects, and a ventricle, a chamber which pumps blood out of the heart.

The right atrium receives blood that has been depleted of oxygen and is loaded with carbon dioxide and other waste products. This blood is passed to the right ventricle. The right ventricle pumps the blood out of the heart and into the lungs to eliminate the carbon dioxide and to pick up oxygen.

Oxygen-rich blood from the lungs then travels to the heart's other collecting chamber, the left atrium, and then passes to the left ventricle. From the left ventricle the blood is pumped to all parts of the body through the circulatory system.

The circulatory system begins at the heart and lungs, and carries the body's nutrients in the blood through arteries, arterioles (small arteries), and capillaries (minute blood vessels), and then through venules (small veins) and veins and back to the heart itself. During its round trip circulation the blood also picks up waste products from the cells of the body to be eliminated through the kidney or lungs.

The pumping action of the heart is controlled by a natural pacemaker, a small bundle of highly specialized cells that generate the electrical impulses necessary for coordinated contractions of the heart. When the heart relaxes, blood flows in as a result of the change in pressure. The valves that allow blood from the right atrium to flow to the right ventricle are open. At this time, the impulse to contract has reached both atria, helping to move the blood to the ventricles.

When the ventricular muscle receives the impulse to contract, the valves between both atria and ventricles are closed by the pressure and the blood is forced out of the heart and to the lungs from the right ventricle and to the body from the left ventricle.

A disease condition develops when the normal flow of blood through the heart and to the body is impeded, when something goes wrong with the heart's pacemaker, or when the blood that supplies nutrients to the heart itself is blocked.

This disease is referred to as cardiovascular (*cardio*—heart and *vascular*—blood vessel) disease. It may damage the brain, the heart, the kidneys or other organs and tissues of the body.

Some of the most vital tissues in the body are perhaps the endocrine glandular system. These are tiny structures composed of groups of highly specialized cells having the ability to secrete hormones that regulate systems necessary for life to continue. The work they perform therefore is vital to the body. Examples are: the parathyroid gland, the adrenal glands and the islet cells of Langerhans in the pancreas.

The retinal membranes of the eyes, although not glandular structures, are commonly affected by cardiovascular disease. Atherosclerosis, thrombosis, emboli and hemorrhagic events can cause loss of blood supply to the retina, and therefore loss of vision.

These structures are anatomically small. The arterioles bringing nutrients and oxygen are very tiny, as are the venules removing metabolic waste products.

A small amount of adherent fatty material might not cause downstream blood supply to vary substantially in a large-caliber artery located elsewhere in the body. Tissue nutrient supply would not be affected enough to cause trouble.

On the other hand, a small but vital group of highly specialized cells such as those comprising the cortex of the adrenal gland is supplied by the small bore arterioles. A tiny, hair-like blood vessel does not have much inside diameter to lose. A small amount of cholesterol or fat can profoundly reduce the blood flow to these cells, and cause critical changes in the body's chemical balance. Wild swings in blood pressure, water retention, heart strain and other abnormal changes can result.

Probably the major underlying condition leading to cardio-vascular disease is atherosclerosis, also known as hardening of the arteries. This degenerative disease, in time, can narrow or block arteries in the heart, brain and other parts of the body. It may begin early in life.

The linings of the arteries become thickened and roughened by deposits of fat, cholesterol, fibrin (a clotting material), cellular debris and calcium.

As this buildup on the inner walls becomes hard and thick, arteries lose their ability to expand and contract. The blood moves with difficulty through the narrowed artery channels. This makes it easier for a clot to form that will block the channel (lumen) and deprive the heart, brain and other organs of a necessary blood supply. In such a situation, how can dilator drugs possibly be effective?

When a complete blockage occurs in a vessel to the brain, the result may be a cerebral thrombosis, a form of stroke. Based on what is known, scientists admit the relationship between the amount of cholesterol and saturated fats in the bloodstream, and coronary artery disease—a blockage of the arteries that supply blood to the heart muscle itself.

The body manufactures its own cholesterol, and scientists have evidence that a diet high in cholesterol and saturated fats will raise cholesterol levels in the blood and contribute to atherosclerosis. Americans consume 40 to 50% of our total caloric intake as fat. It would be wise to reduce this figure to 20%, and thereby lower the risk of heart disease and stroke.

SIGNS OF HEART ABNORMALITIES

The most commonly noted signs of early heart diseases are probably erratic heart rhythms. The heart may speed up abnormally to rates between 100 beats per minute to over 200 beats per minute. This may last for varying lengths of times and can cause serious degrees of anxiety, shortness of breath and lightheadedness or fainting. The heartbeat may be regular, but fast. It can also be irregular, with no pattern.

Pain, usually in the center of the chest, may be present. The pain can move up the neck and involve the teeth or jaw.

It can radiate to the upper back. It can move down the left or the right arm.

The pain usually subsides in a short time, but may begin again following stress or physical activity.

Do not ignore these warning signs and symptoms. Seek medical attention, and if your doctor does not advise a stress electrocardiogram test (taken while the patient walks on a treadmill, or pedals a bicycle) request it. If he cannot do it, ask him to refer you to a clinic with that capability.

The usual electrocardiogram, taken with the patient resting or lying on a table, can miss important early diagnostic information. This, however, is the usual type of electrocardiogram test given by most doctors.

To narrow the possibility of error, a stress electrocardiogram is necessary. Even this test is not fool-proof, but it lowers the chance of error greatly.

THROMBOSIS

In 1899 Welch defined a thrombus as "a solid mass or plug formed in the living heart or vessels from constituents of the blood." The definition is still valid.

To this day medical science does not know the precise mechanism involved in the formation of thromboses, despite extensive research. As an idea of the over-all importance of thrombosis it is estimated that diseases complicated or caused by thromboembolism occur about three times more frequently than cancer. (*Cecil Textbook of Medicine,* Beeson, McDermott and Wyngaarden, 1979, W.B. Sanders Company, Philadelphia.)

The consensus of medical opinion is that all thrombi are initiated by platelets sticking to the endothelial surface of the vessel's interior. These platelets trigger the conversion of fibrinogen to fibrin, which forms a net-like structure to contain more platelets. The initial stimulus can be endothelial damage, caused by high blood pressure, chemicals or toxins, or deficiencies of certain nutrients. Fats and lipids infiltrate the thrombus and eventually calcium will infiltrate the plaque formation and the vessel wall.

Recent studies from Finland suggest that the trace metal selenium is protective of the cardiovascular system. A seven year study of 11,000 people from two countries of eastern Finland known for their high incidence of cardiovascular mortality was conducted. These counties also happened to have very low soil selenium.

The relationship between selenium levels in the blood serum and heart disease was highly significant. When serum selenium fell below 45 micrograms per liter, all patients had high risk of myocardial infarction compared to a control group of patients whose serum contained more than 45 micrograms per liter.

When serum selenium fell below 34 micrograms per liter the risk of coronary heart disease and cardiovascular disease death was much higher than at levels between 35 and 44 micrograms per liter.

Since selenium is a necessary part of the glutathione peroxidase enzyme reaction, inadequate dietary selenium might reduce the peroxidation of this enzyme and lead to an accumulation of lipid peroxides, which in turn, can injure the arterial endothelial lining. There is evidence now linking selenium deficiency to increased platelet aggregation. (Saonenm J.T., et al, *1982 Association Between Cardiovascular Death, Myocardial Infarction and Selenium In a Matched Pair Longitudinal Study,* Lancet, 2:175-179.)

Kakkar's study of 469 consecutive patients aged forty or over, undergoing elective surgery, revealed that 28% developed deep leg vein thrombosis. Older patients having major operations have an incidence of more than 50%. The highest risk is in patients having reconstructive or total hip replacement surgery.

SIGNS OF THROMBOSIS

Thrombosis can occur gradually or suddenly. The vein can be felt under the skin. It is tender and painful, and may be inflamed and reddened. As the process creeps along the vessel wall, a reddish streaking can be seen. This can become infected, and a patient can develop a fever.

In the veins that lie deep beneath the surface, the pain may be minimal or absent entirely. One cannot see inflammatory changes. The limb may feel spongy or "doughy" when squeezed or massaged. The leg will swell somewhat, but it may be necessary to measure the circumference with a tape measure to demonstrate early changes. Flexion of the foot sometimes causes pain in the calf of the affected leg.

Doppler ultrasonic examination and plethysmography are non-invasive methods of testing that will confirm the diagnosis.

Should a clot break away from the thrombotic leg vein, it can move with the blood flow, eventually to lodge in the lung. This condition is called pulmonary embolism, a serious life-threatening catastrophe. I feel that with proper supplementation (vitamins A, C, E, selenium and other vitamins and minerals) and physiotherapy and exercise therapy, this condition can be reduced dramatically. Pulmonary embolism should be a medical rarity.

Unfortunately, the reverse is true. Next to pneumonia, it is the most common acute pulmonary lesion seen in hospitalized patients. Had these patients undergone chelation therapy, the majority would most likely have avoided hospitalization. Those few who might have been hospitalized would have had their stays shortened because conventional drugs and procedures would have worked better in less time. The chance of pulmonary embolism would be drastically reduced, if seen at all.

Nearly one-fourth of all people killed by cardiovascular disease are under age sixty-five, a needless waste of life. Nearly one million people (975,550) in 1979 died of cardiovascular disease. This computes to being 51% of all deaths in the United States that year. Atherosclerosis contributed to many of the 719,200 heart attack and stroke deaths in 1979.

How do American physicians cope with this onslaught?

Unfortunately, when the doctor suspects, after preliminary examination, that a patient has early disease of the heart or blood vessels, the first treatment is usually no treatment. In the terminology of the profession, this is called "watchful expectancy." The doctor will tell the patient, "Let's watch it for a month," or "I'll want to check you again in a year."

I have had patients with severe occlusive vascular disease who have been told to do nothing, take things easy, and return in a year to eighteen months when the condition is *bad enough to operate.* One gentleman in his forties could not walk two blocks because of pain in his lower back and legs. He had become impotent. He could barely get through his work day, consisting of supervising a work crew for the water company. He was told his condition, occlusion of the lower aorta at its bifurcation, was not yet *bad enough* to operate. The doctor referred him to a vascular surgeon who concurred with the other physican, and added there was no other way to treat the condition except surgically, inserting a synthetic graft in place of the plugged-up portion of the aorta.

This patient was chelated with EDTA. Without surgery he has made a complete recovery. His impotency has disappeared and his energy level is better than it has been in ten years. He has no limitation on the distance he can now walk.

The most recent figures available that tell the alarming story of heart and blood vessel disease are contained in The American Heart Association publication, *Heart Facts 1982.*

Item: 41,290,000 Americans have one or more forms of heart or blood vessel disease. This is roughly one out of every five people.

Item: Stroke afflicts 1,780,000 Americans.

Item: As many as 1.5 million Americans may have a heart attack this year and about 550,000 will die.'

Item: High blood pressure (hypertension) afflicts an estimated 35,520,000 American adults.

Item: 1,820,000 adults and 100,000 children in America have rheumatic heart disease.

Item: The economic cost of cardiovascular disease will amount to an estimated $50.7 billion in 1982. This breaks down to $12,270.50 as the average cost per patient.

The first three paragraphs of *Heart Facts* outline the great impact of this illness on the American public.

"Together these diseases kill more Americans than all other causes of death combined. Each year nearly one million deaths are attributed to these diseases. That's more deaths than are caused by cancer, accidents, pneumonia, influenza and so on—all combined."

"The major underlying cause that has been associated with the high incidence of these diseases is atherosclerosis, a buildup of fatty deposits within the walls of the arteries that restricts, and sometimes blocks completely, the flow of blood to the vital organs in the body. Studies implicate high cholesterol levels in the blood, high blood pressure and cigarette smoking as contributors to atherosclerosis."

"Medical science has made important advances in the prevention and treatment of these diseases and has, thereby, found ways to reduce the risk of heart disease and stroke and to prevent the buildup of atherosclerosis by lowering high blood pressure, discouraging cigarette smoking, and by lowering the amount of cholesterol and saturated fats in the diet."

"The AHA is a nonprofit voluntary health agency, supported solely by private contributions and not government tax dollars, whose mission is to reduce early death and disability from heart disease, stroke and related disorders. It does this by supporting research, professional and public education and community service programs."

If the American Heart Association takes its mission seriously, and wants to improve its batting average in reducing early death and disability from heart disease, stroke and related disorders, the organization is ignoring a most important treatment contribution, EDTA chelation.

Doctors in the United States using EDTA chelation treatment have been successfully reversing the effects of heart disease since the 1950s. It would seem that the AHA could by this time test chelation procedure themselves, and publish their findings.

Chelation Therapy And Cardiovascular Disease 41

6
Chelation Therapy
And Atherosclerosis

The word *atheroma* is derived from the Greek word meaning *porridge*. Early investigators used the word to describe the fatty pebble-like appearance of the atheromatous artery's interior. This disease was found routinely when Egyptian mummies were examined. From that time until the present, traditional medicine has not been able to slow, or prevent atherosclerosis.

The disease commonly invades large and medium sized arteries. Those most regularly affected include the aorta, iliac, femoral, coronary, carotid and cerebral arteries.

Estimated annual costs for treatment of atherosclerotic disease in the United States is $52 billion. For the individual patient, costs will reach more than $12,000 per annum, or $1,000.00 per month. These costs reflect only after-the-fact care, that is, dollars required for control.

The atherosclerotic plaque is comprised of a mixture of cells (mostly of smooth muscle origin), connective tissue (elastin and collagen), and lipids (cholesterol, triglycerides and phospholipids) inside and outside the cells of the plaque.

This messy, gooey sludge is infiltrated with calcium as it

develops. Eventually the whole mess becomes hardened. Now, it has the consistency of slag.

The atherosclerotic process, namely, the deposition of the various components, the changing from a sludge-like stage to the hardened slag stage, goes on simultaneously in many arteries in different locations of the body.

Surgery on one area of the arterial system that is too advanced to permit normal organ function is treatment too little and too late. Nothing is usually done for the remaining arteries that need preventive care. This would be too costly. The risk to the patient would be unacceptable, for morbidity and mortality rates would soar.

Blood pressure elevation can lead to the development of atherosclerosis. Systolic blood pressure greater than 160 millimeters of mercury, or diastolic blood pressure greater than 95 millimeters of mercury causes a five-fold increased risk of coronary heart disease compared to people with normal blood pressure.

High blood pressure is the greatest risk factor overall for disease in people older than forty-five years. Obesity, and increased intake of fats and refined sugar, and lack of exercise are risks of major importance.

Studies made by the Department of Pathology, United States Army, revealed that approximately 40% of autopsies conducted on Korean casualties exhibited "significant" occlusion of the arteries.

Using the same protocol on the same number (3,000) of soldiers killed in Vietnam, 70% were found to have this condition. The average age of both groups was 21.8 years.

This insidious chronic degenerative occlusive vascular disease (called atherosclerosis) is rapidly becoming an epidemic in this country. By these findings we can conclude that "significant" occlusion, that is, plugging, occluding or narrowing at least 65% on the anterior space in the arteries takes about twenty years.

In the field of cardiovascular disease, medical thinking has finally realized that atherosclerotic disease does not suddenly become established inside a patient's arteries. The process is subtle. There is a lengthy time lag before the diagnosis is made. It is characterized by a gradual build-up of fatty sludge that clogs the vessel sufficiently to eventually produce problems and lead to the diagnosis. These progressive events are more descriptively labeled *atherogenesis.*

It is difficult to diagnose because the patient is generally free of obvious symptoms and physicians are not looking for early disease. They have been trained to find a reason for the patient's complaints, an after-the-fact approach.

Doctor Iwao M. Moriyama, Chief of the Office of Health Statistics Analysis, in a report released by the United States Department of Health, Education and Welfare, pointed out that in the period 1939-1960, the crude death rate dropped from 17.2 to 9.5 per 1,000 population. Current figures, however, indicate that trend now appears to have leveled off during the recorded decade 1950-1960. Doctor Moriyama expressed concern about the stationary 1950-1960 trend:

"The failure to experience a decline in the mortality during this period is unexpected in view of the intensified attack on medical problems in the postwar years. In this setting it would seem reasonable to expect further reductions in mortality. On the other hand, the possible adverse effects on mortality or radioactive fallout, air pollution and other man-made hazards cannot be completely ignored. If the leveling off of the death rates has resulted from failure to prevent deaths that are preventable, this is of public health significance."

According to Doctor William H. Stewart, formerly of the Division of Public Health Methods, United States Public Health Service, there has been a dramatic curtailment of acute infectious diseases leading to death and a gradual rise in mortality due to chronic disorders. For the most part, the overall downward trend has been checked by the current trends among the chronic disorders. Despite intensified research, heart disease, cancer and stroke continue to rate overwhelmingly as the leading causes of death in the United States at the present time. In 1963, these three groups of disorders, collectively, accounted for 71% of all deaths in the nation.

HOW CHELATION WORKS TO REVERSE THE PROBLEM

The atherosclerotic process is not limited to the coronary arteries. Any artery can be affected, but the initial event is the same: injury to the delicate inner lining of the artery wall. High blood pressure, smoking, viruses, allergies, carbon monoxide, elevations in the cholesterol, uric acid, triglycerides, metabolic toxins from malfunctioning organs, bacterial infection of the artery wall and probably many other mechanisms can injure the intimal lining.

If we affect a re-opening of the arteries all over the body, then the organs should benefit. They do, and blood chemistries of all the organs have shown this improvement in all of our patients over the years. As calcium is removed by EDTA, the magnetic holding of fats and cholesterol to the calcium in the vessel wall is no more. The former close association of the plaque material is lost, they become *unglued.* The vessels now have more open space for the blood to flow through, and the arteries are now able to deliver much needed nutrients and precious oxygen. The veins, also carrying more blood, are able to remove metabolic cellular wastes more efficiently.

Robert W. Eissler, Ph.D., M.D., Director, Specialized Center of Research in Atherosclerosis, University of Chicago, writing in *Modern Concepts of Cardiovascular Disease,* volume XLVI, page 27, 1977, states that "a growing body of evidence indicates that the process of atherosclerosis is almost completely preventable and that it is substantially reversible."

When a patient completes chelation therapy vascular testing (plethysmography and occulocerebrovasculometry), stress treadmill tests and blood chemistries show the vessels to be opened inside.

It is unlikely that sudden severe occlusion will reassert itself in the short run. Rather, it is more likely that many years of the worst possible lifestyle would be necessary to put the patient in jeopardy once again.

I have yet to see a patient who purposely tries to wreck his health to that extent. The majority of patients are happy and thankful they have been able to reverse the degenerative process. They improve their lifestyle. They want to maintain their improvement.

7
Chelation Therapy And High Blood Pressure

People with greatly elevated blood pressure commonly have symptoms of dizziness, shortness of breath, headache and blurred vision. In mild to moderate blood pressure elevation, there may be no symptoms.

The diastolic or resting heart pressure is the second number of the blood pressure reading. In younger patients with diastolic pressures of 110 millimeters of mercury or higher, headaches in the morning are common. Breathlessness produced by easy effort, such as slow walking is common. The patient may notice pulsation of neck veins which may also be swollen and distended. A clicking or roaring or ringing in the ears is a frequent finding.

High blood pressure patients commonly complain of frequent need to urinate after they have gone to bed for the night, even though kidney function may be normal. Hypertension commonly occurs as the result of local ischemia (loss of oxygen carried by the blood) which has resulted from atheromatous narrowing (occlusion) of an artery in the brain, heart, or lower limbs.

As the pressure continues its abnormal rise, death or damage to the heart, brain or kidneys is likely. The heart will enlarge, kidneys begin to fail, and uremia is present. Stroke is common.

These patients commonly range in age from forty to seventy. Their blood pressure is above 110 millimeters mercury (diastolic). Systolic pressures (the first numbers of the blood pressure reading), range from 130 to 170 or more.

In a thirty-five year old man with a normal blood pressure of 120/80, the risk of death over the next twenty years would double if his presure were 142/90. That risk increases 2.2 times at 142/95. At 152/95, the twenty year mortality risk is 2.5 times.

LDL cholesterol is directly and independently associated with cardiovascular risks. HDL cholesterol, on the other hand, appears to offer protection.

Aerobic exercise, liver function and supplementation with digestive enzymes and selected amino acids can enable the patient to favorably adjust the HDL/LDL ratio, and hence, reduce cardiovascular disease risk. Dietary modification of saturated fats and cholesterol is an important step to include, and make permament, in the patient's lifestyle.

In addition to selenium deficiencies, these patients usually have reduced magnesium and potassium. Protein and microscopic bleeding are commonly found in the urine. Damage to the retinal membranes of the eye results from leaking arterioles. Flame hemorrhages, cotton wool exudates, atrioventricular nicking and scaling of the arterioles can be seen on examination. As blood pressure rises, the arterioles constrict and eventually give way to the pressure. Leakage occurs and this seeing membrane (retina) swells. Visual loss results.

Similar damage occurs in the brain. Patients with abnormally high blood pressure and increasingly severe headaches can progress eventually to impairment of brain function and stupor. The brain swells as plasma leaks out from the arterioles.

Abrupt onset of neurological signs such as numbness, nausea, vomiting, loss of muscle function in the face, arm, or leg followed by unconsciousness, signifies the onset of bleeding inside the skull. This is a stroke.

8
Chelation Therapy And Irregular Heart Rhythm

Thousands of electrocardiogram tracings of patients' heart activity before, during and after chelation with EDTA have demonstrated that this treatment is remarkably beneficial to cardiac arrhythmias (abnormal heart rhythms).

Sinus bradycardia, sinus tachycardia, sinoatrial block, artrial extrasystoles, atrial fibrillation and flutter and ventricular tachycardia respond well to EDTA treatment. The heartbeat becomes smooth, regular and more efficient and the P-R interval shortens. On the treadmill, ST segment depression is reversed. These findings are being published by our group at McDonagh Medical Center.

Several mechanisms of action operating simultaneously are responsible for the outstanding improvement in cardiac rhythm.

Excess calcium and lipids are removed from heart muscle cells. Membranes of the cell wall, mitochondria and nucleus are able to revitalize and repair themselves under the influence of EDTA. Normal enzyme chemistry of the heart (and body) cells is enhanced and restored. Improved circulation of the nourishing blood vessels brings selenium, potassium, vitamins, oxygen and other necessary nutrients in adequate (increased) amounts to the working heart muscle. Metabolic wastes inside heart muscle cells that were unable to exit the cells expeditiously due to faulty membrane biochemistry are now eliminated.

When the cell membranes normalize, nutrients can enter, and the normal function is reestablished. Wastes are passed out through the cell membrane, to be picked up by the reactivated circulation, and eventually eliminated from the body.

Patients taking medication to control their disease have been able to reduce these drug dosages. The majority can eventually eliminate drugs.

EDTA chelation, therefore, enables heart drugs to work more effectively. This is the reason a patient can reduce drug dosage and at the same time improve his heart and his health.

Cardiovascular drug dosages usually become less effective the longer the patient takes them. Dosages must be increased or additional drugs added in order to maintain the same degree of control. It is not unusual to see a new patient taking seven or eight drugs several times daily, complain of increasing symptoms of cardiovascular disease. To reverse this trend while eliminating the disease, no other treatment is as important as chelation with EDTA. In fact, no other treatment has this capability.

9

Chelation Therapy
And Stroke

An artery feeding the brain gradually crusts over inside until one day it becomes plugged completely.

A small balloon-like swelling appears on the side of an artery in the brain and eventually enlarges as a result of increased blood pressure. Ultimately it will rupture and bleeding into brain tissue will occur. Or possibly a blood clot enters an artery that feeds the brain. Its progress gradually slows as the vessel branches and becomes smaller. Suddenly it cannot pass any farther, and the vessel is completely occluded.

Four people are riding in the front seat of a pickup truck that skids into a ditch during a snow storm. The truck rests on its side, and the person on the bottom has his neck compressed against the windowsill by the weight of his companions above him.

All of the examples describe a common American malady—the birth of a stroke.

A stroke is the end result of sudden deprivation of oxygenated blood to the brain. In 1979, 169,000 people died of stroke in this country. There are one-half million new stroke victims each year. Some 1,780,000 persons have survived a stroke in this country, and have some form of residual functional loss ranging from slight to serious.

The very same set of circumstances that causes occlusion in the coronary arteries is at work in the arteries that bring blood to the brain. It is the same process in a different artery. Once again, atherosclerosis is the culprit. If blood is suddenly shut off, the brain cannot function, just as the heart cannot function if its coronary blood supply is lost. The only thing that changes is diagnostic terminology. In one case it is a heart attack, in the other it is a stroke.

Cerebral thrombosis, a common form of stroke, occurs when one of the arteries supplying blood to a section of the brain is blocked by a clot (thrombus) that forms inside the artery. This can happen readily in an artery that has been damaged by our old enemy, atherosclerosis.

A cerebral embolism, another form of stroke, can be caused by a wandering clot (embolus) that breaks loose from an atherosclerotic plaque and flows downstream with the blood. An artery becomes smaller inside and out the farther it travels from its source.

Veins, on the other hand, generally become larger the farther they get from their point of origin. This enables them to carry more blood back to the heart.

As it reaches out to the brain to deliver nutrient-laden blood, an artery is characterized by many branches. At some point along the inside of that artery, a clot will be too large to pass the narrowing channel. When it wedges tight, no blood will pass and a stroke ensues.

The term *cerebro vascular occlusion* describes the previous two examples (*cerebro,* meaning brain, and *vascular,* meaning blood vessel).

On the other hand, a cerebral hemorrhage differs from the above examples because it occurs as a result of a rupture of an atherosclerotic artery in the brain. Bleeding into the surrounding brain tissue occurs. The flood of blood reduces blood flow and pressure. No blood can travel past the site of vessel rupture. Brain tissue downstream is deprived of its supply, and those brain cells cannot function. In addition, continued bleeding from the ruptured vessel can put pressure on surrounding brain tissue and cause mild to severe loss of function.

Hemorrhage from an artery in the brain can also be caused by head injury or by a ruptured aneurysm. Aneurysms are pouches that balloon out from the weakened artery wall. Most of these are associated with high blood pressure. Pressure causes the wall of the aneurysm to pouch out farther and farther. The wall becomes thinner as the pouch gets larger. Eventually a rupture results.

The same mechanism operates if too much air is pumped into a bicycle tire. An egg-shaped blob appears on the side of the tire (aneurysm) which grows larger. The wall of the pouch gets thinner as the pouch becomes larger. Eventually, if air pressure is not reduced, the blob will rupture (blow out) and the tire will go flat.

If an aneurysm ruptures in the brain, a stroke results. After effects of stroke vary with the amount and location of brain tissue that is denied its blood supply. The patient can be totally paralyzed, or perhaps deprived of the use of an arm, or leg or facial muscles on one side of the body. Some victims cannot speak. Some cannot walk. Many have no control over their bowels or bladder, and require constant nursing care. Stroke damage to the brain may affect the senses, behavior patterns, memory and thought patterns. Some patients have visual changes.

The size of the vessel that occludes is important, too. If a large caliber vessel at the base of the brain suddenly occludes, death usually occurs quite rapidly. At the periphery, the end of the vascular tree in the brain, the vessels are much smaller, and therefore deliver nourishment and oxygen to smaller segments of brain tissue. If one of these occludes, a smaller amount of brain tissue is lost, and the chances for survival are good.

If you must have a stroke, the best thing is to have a small clot plug the tiny vessel in the outermost portion of the brain, right?

Wrong! Once established, any clot can grow fantastically,

sometimes occluding many branches of the artery. This process is called clot propagation.

In this country, we have a rather ineffective and discouraging track record in preventing strokes and reversing "permanent damage" that has resulted from a stroke. When brain tissue downstream from an occluded artery is denied its blood supply, the tissue cannot operate normally. Function quits immediately. Tissue begins to die after a time, and changes that result are permanent.

Of those unfortunate patients who have their first stroke, fifteen out of one hundred will be killed as a result of this cerebral vascular accident. Eighty-five survive, but half of these will be totally and permanently disabled.

When the vessel that services brain tissue in control of speech, or hearing, or vision, or muscular functions of the arms, legs, urinary bladder, or any other body part is unable to supply oxygen and nutrients, that function is affected. The patient cannot talk, hear, see, or have use of the arms, legs, or the urinary bladder.

Stroke is usually thought of as a disease of the elderly, and proportionally there are more strokes in those over the age of sixty. It is not unusual however, to see younger people with the unmistakable aftereffects of stroke. In every community there are cases of stroke survivors with permanent loss of arms or legs, memory or the ability to think.

These changes can be reversed through EDTA chelation therapy.

We commonly see such patients in their thirties and forties. The medical literature reports an increasing number of strokes each year in those under fifteen years of age.

The umbrella term used to describe the collection of signs and symptoms that may occur prior to a stroke is TIA, or *transient ischemic attack*. Approximately 60 to 70% of stroke victims have no warning signs. Of the remainder, they may have such TIA signs or symptoms such as:

• Temporary dizziness, with a tendency to lean to one side.

• Disturbance of vision, or transient blindness.

- Nausea, vomiting, fainting, falling.
- Unusual numbness or tingling of face, arm, hand, leg, foot.
- Weakness or paralysis in an arm or leg that may last for a period of time, then disappear.
- Loss of urinary bladder control.
- Loss of hearing or speech.
- Inability to think, loss of awareness.
- Any one or combination of the above.

TIAs are more common in elderly patients, probably because they have lived long enough to develop significant occlusive vascular disease. The biochemistry of the aging brain has been studied, and factors other than circulation of the brain have been found that contribute to stroke and senility.

Neurohormones and neuroenzymes that make oxygen available to the brain cells begin to malfunction. Oxygen and nutrients cannot be properly utilized by the cells. Functional efficiency declines. The cells must make do with less. Sooner or later function slips, and we say grandpa is getting confused, senile, old.

The chemical efficiency of the cell is unable to continue as before, and loss of function is the result. The patient cannot think quickly. He cannot hear or see as well as he did a few years ago. His organs and muscles do not work properly.

The immune system gradually loses efficiency. Injuries and infections from bacteria, viruses, fungi take longer than usual to be overcome.

Irritation of the arterial endothelium that lines the inside walls comprising the lumen—by physical, chemical or immunological means—can cause the vessel to contract and shut off the flow of blood to the brain. Chronic use of tobacco, caffeine, alcohol, refined sugar and flour can aggravate the artery by chemical means. Lead, cadmium, drugs, insecticides and other toxic chemicals can cause similar damage. The circular coats of the artery—when thus stimulated abnormally—contract, and shut off the flow of blood. The mechanism is similar to closing a duffle bag. When the strings are pulled, the opening becomes progressively smaller. When the artery is completely shut down, it is bad news for cells downstream.

The American Heart Association states that stroke treatment may include surgery, drugs, hospital care and rehabilitation. In those cases where the blockage has occured in the arteries of the neck, surgery called carotid endarterectomy may be used to remove the artherosclerotic plaque.

To perform carotid endarterectomy, the surgeon must slit the artery in the neck, opening it along the area that is most occluded. He then removes the occluding sludge-like material, and sews shut the incision in the artery. The tissues of the neck and skin are next stitched closed. Several inches of slimy material having the consistency of an unripe banana, are removed from the inside of the artery. Sometimes the occlusive material becomes hardened with minerals, fibrin, platelets and cholesterol.

Carotid endarterectomy can prevent a stroke, and if a patient's carotids are dangerously occluded, he should have the operation. It is of paramount importance to remember that this procedure removes only a few inches of occlusive material. It cannot clean those arteries at the base of the brain, or inside the brain itself. They are not within reach of the scalpel. For the most part, these arteries are surgically untreatable. The approach itself would cause significant brain damage.

A neurosurgeon's approach to a vessel with a small aneurism is to tie off the vessel, preventing a rupture later on. Again, tissue downstream will suffer from nutrient deprivation and oxygen loss.

The AHA states that for cases where a blood vessel has been blocked by a clot, anti-clotting drugs may be used to prevent new clots from forming, or to prevent an existing clot from getting bigger (clot propagation). The association does not address the question of what to do with the clot already formed. Will these measures remove it?

Dr. William E. Evans, M.D., Clinical Professor of Surgery,

Ohio State University, speaking at a recent vascular medicine symposium held in Sarasota, Florida, informed the assembled physicians that TIAs are a surgical problem. He also stated that patients who have had a stroke should not undergo surgery because the operation will make the condition worse. He said there is no increase in blood flow to the brain following carotid endarterectomy in these patients.

As to preventing a stroke, the AHA is vague. The best way to prevent a stroke, they say, is to reduce those factors that cause the stroke in the first place. Many strokes can be prevented if high blood pressure is diagnosed and controlled. Another important way to reduce the risk of stroke is to identify and treat little strokes or TIAs. Many major strokes are preceded by these early warning signals, which may occur days, weeks, or months before the more severe event. Prompt medical or surgical attention to these symptoms may prevent a fatal or disabling stroke. No argument here.

But what of the 60 to 70% of stroke victims who have no warning signs or symptoms?

The accepted prevention and treatment, therefore, is after the fact. Once a patient has symptoms or has a stroke, something should be done, according to the AHA.

All of us must keep in mind that when symptoms occur, the disease is already in a dangerously advanced state. The coming major catastrophe will suddenly strike the patient down. Treatment then has little if any chance of bringing that patient back to normal function.

Physicians must maintain a healthy suspicion of vascular disease in stroke-prone people. A few blood tests, a good history and physical examination and plethsysmographic tracings (arterial pulse volume recordings) should be done. All of these can be done in the doctor's office.

RISK FACTORS OF THE
STROKE-PRONE PATIENT

Fortunately, most risk factors for stroke can be reduced or eliminated if the patient desires and perseveres. High blood pressure control (or elimination) reduces the risk of stroke.

Heart disease increases the risk of stroke. The failing

pump-action of the heart is a source of emboli, clots that form in the heart. They could enter the arteries that supply the brain and cause a stroke. Good management of heart disease would necessitate EDTA chelation treatment. The risk in this case would be greatly reduced if not eliminated entirely.

Diabetes mellitus. Chelation does an excellent job in reducing the vasculitis of diabetes. Circulation is restored throughout the body and stroke risk is minimized.

Some risk factors cannot be changed, however. The risk of stroke in men is greater than the risk for women. Women smokers who take oral contraceptives have an increased risk of stroke.

The risk of death and disability from stroke is much greater among black Americans than among whites, pro- bably because of the greater prevalence of hypertension among blacks. EDTA can reduce this problem greatly, simp- ly by reducing blood pressure.

By cleaning the lumen (inside space) of the arteries, and removing the slag and sludge, the space available for the blood to occupy is increased. When the space increases, the pressure drops. Eventually normal blood pressure prevails.

There are some patients who have other causes for their blood pressure elevation. These cases generally respond to the normalization of the cellular membranes, increased cellular oxygen and the nutrient support that is part and parcel of the chelation treatment method.

In summary, strokes are caused by the same factors that cause reduction in blood flow in other vascular diseases such as heart attacks, gangrene, and so on. The symptoms are completely different because of the effect of circulatory loss on the downstream tissue (brain). Symptoms vary depend- ing upon the area of brain involved. Remember, symptoms happen after the disease process had progressed sufficient- ly. Many people (including some physicians) fail to distin- guish between symptoms and the disease that causes them.

The reasons EDTA chelation is so successful in chronic diseases is the fact that all of these conditions have an abnormal vascular component that the usual medical treatment cannot help. Herein lies the opportunity for prevention of these devastating diseases. Physicians must look for the very earliest signs of circulatory embarrassment long before signs and symptoms of disease are apparent. Like the distant early warning radar system (DEW line) that serves to protect our country in case of a sneak air or missile attack, we must strive to be better medical detectives.

During my medical training, we were taught that if a patient survived a stroke, a short period of time was available to rehabilitate him. That period might be several months, or might be as long as a year. Physiotherapy, gait training exercises and speech therapy were prescribed. The patient was treated aggressively. Some degree of improvement was noted. Sometimes it was small, indeed.

After the patient had completed one year of therapy following his stroke, it was thought no further improvement could be expected. This is still the unspoken rule today.

These are the people you see in wheelchairs. Nursing homes are loaded with them. Those who are fortunate in having someone at home who is willing to care for them are frequently seen shuffling pitifully along the sidewalk with the aid of crutches, canes. Many require four-legged walkers. Some cannot use their hands or arms and are frequently seen in their wheelchairs with one arm in a sling. Residual facial paralysis is common. The ability to control the urinary bladder may not return, and the patient constantly wets his clothing.

Talking is difficult for some, impossible for others. Thinking and emotional response is similarly affected. The patient usually becomes severely depressed and withdrawn.

Many patients become cranky, easily irritated, ill tempered and uncooperative. They have no hope and so they give up on living. They vegetate until they die. They become a burden to themselves and to those who love them.

Because their immune system is depressed by the chronicity of the disease process, they become susceptible to infections. They require increasing amounts of costly medical care.

Stiffened muscles and joints refuse to cooperate when the patient attempts to move about. A fall can result in the fracture of a leg or hip. After the bone has been set, or the hip pinned surgically, pneumonia or congestive heart failure become common killers during the recovery period.

The picture of stroke is dark. Without a doubt, it is bad news.

In the brain the hair-like, thread-sized blood vessels are sandwiched between groups of cells. There are so many of them at the periphery of the cerebral cortex, the cell mass denied oxygenated blood by the occluded vessel can get nourishment from the vessel next door. Needed nutrients ooze from the wall of these tiny vessels.

Waste products, however, are not removed as efficiently, and they increase in amount and concentration. The cells in the area of occlusion thus become toxic, that is, poisoned by their own metabolic waste products. Brain cells become dormant and cease to function. They will ultimately die, but the time period is remarkably long. I am constantly amazed and delighted by the progress made by patients who have reversed post-stroke paralysis and functional loss they have endured for many years.

Chelation with EDTA can change the black, bleak portrait of stroke to one of brightness and sunlight. People who were unable to walk with crutches and walkers have been able to shed them and walk without assistance. Those who have lost their speech impairments, talk normally again. Mental machinery is normalized enabling patients to think correctly and quickly again. Organ systems improve and normalize. Stroke victims come out of their shell, become cheerful, and leave their depression behind. Eyesight improves. Resistance to infectious disease is strengthened. Such recovering stroke victims rarely get ill following completion of chelation treatment. The withered, aged look disappears. In short, these beneficiaries of chelation therapy begin to live normally again. Many of them become stronger and healthier than they were before their stroke.

Many patients forced to retire because of their permanent disability following a stroke have gone back to work. Some have begun new businesses. All have been snatched from the wheelchair or rocking chair and given a lease on unencumbered living. Without chelation with EDTA, would they have had a chance? No chance at all!

The chelation treatment is not specific for stroke. This is perhaps its strongest point. The intravenous method insures simultaneous action throughout the circulatory system. This is a great help to patients, because many have more than one pathological problem operating. The usual approach to a patient with several problems is to treat the worst and tackle the others later. Sometimes minor diagnoses are ignored.

Metabolic stress is not eliminated under these circumstances. First, the body's ability to concentrate its healing ability is lost or compromised. It must be spread very thin to cover several disease processes, and many times it cannot do the job.

As a part of chelation therapy, the intravenous fluid is dripped into a vein—and from that point, circulates through every blood vessel in the body. During its travels, chelating materials, vitamins, trace minerals and other nutrients are supplied to all cells and tissues that need them. Wastes are removed. Organ function improves. Things work better.

When all areas of pathology are addressed, the body can heal itself efficiently and quickly. I am constantly delighted at the ability of the most advanced and critically ill patients to make a rapid comeback, even patients with ten or twelve diagnostic problems, patients who have been bedridden for years. E. Cheraskin, M.D., who heads the research department at McDonagh Medical Center, has told me after checking patient records monthly for more than a year, he found that our average patient has eight diagnostic problems.

Improvements in bodily functions just described for stroke victims are not theoretical or imagined. These results are documented in the case histories of thousands of patients who have undergone chelation with EDTA at McDonagh Medical Center.

It is true that chelation is successful in a great variety of chronic degenerative disease, but in stroke, it is uniquely successful. Many patients can literally be rescued from the grim reaper. They appear lost, withdrawn, depressed before treatment. Their muscles are loose and flabby. Their skin is dried and wrinkled. And their eyes are sunken. They are visibly failing, dying slowly before the eyes of their own families.

Ideally, the easiest stroke to treat is the one that never happens. Early diagnostic testing can uncover dangerous vascular conditions that will lead to stroke. The stroke-prone patient might have had some early warnings. This is the case with 30 to 40% of our patients.

If no sign or unexplained symptom becomes evident, the problem can be discovered nevertheless by means of noninvasive testing. Treatment intervention now will prevent stroke, and it will reverse atherosclerosis, thereby removing the risk of subsequent strokes or other vascular accidents.

A case that illustrates this is that of C.I., a forty-nine year old lady who came to our clinic one afternoon six years ago. She had been awakened in the middle of the night by a severe headache. The pain would not respond to aspirin or other home remedies, and she could not sleep for the rest of the night. The patient dialed her doctor at five in the morning and arranged to meet him at the hospital. After examining her, he made a diagnosis of migraine headache. The doctor prescribed a narcotic, and told the patient to return home, take the medication, and she would probably sleep four or five hours. He expected her to awaken pain-free.

The narcotic dulled the pain, but she could not sleep. After an hour or two she noted the left side of her face had developed a "funny" numb feeling. Looking into a mirror, she found the facial muscles on that side would not move when she smiled.

She notified the doctor again and went to his office. A new

diagnosis of Bell's palsy was made, a condition resulting from a previous viral infection that affects the nerves to those muscles. The doctor gave her a steroid injection, and applied heat to the face.

Shortly after returning home, she noted weakness developing in the left arm and leg. She then drove to our clinic, a distance of about 150 miles.

Testing revealed occlusion of the carotid arteries, especially the internal carotid artery. EDTA chelation therapy was started immediately. Within four hours, she stated that her numbness was improved. By the fifth treatment it had left, and her hand grip strength had noticeably improved.

By the end of the month this lady had completely recovered. She had taken sixteen treatments. We see her every six to nine months. She has had no further trouble.

Probably the worst case of stroke paralysis that I can recall is that of Dr. W. P.

This man, in his late fifties, had suffered a series of vascular accidents fourteen years before. He had been an alcoholic and smoked three or more packages of unfiltered cigarettes daily prior to his first stroke. His history indicated two strokes and at least one heart attack. He was semi-comatose and was deteriorating rapidly.

The patient was hospitalized in another state. His wife called a physician in Kansas City, requesting the patient be hospitalized there for treatment.

One hot summer night this doctor called, asking if I would consult on the case, and manage EDTA chelation therapy for him. He had heard about the treatment, but had no experience with it.

Treatment was begun. EDTA dosages were small. Progress was slow. The patient had been unable to maintain his weight, and was literally skin and bones. Both shoulders, sides and hips exhibited multiple pressure ulcerations (bed sores). He was curled up into a fetal position. He could not feed himself, and could not swallow properly. He could not control his bladder or his bowels. He could make no sound except an occasional groan or mumble. His food and supplemental nutrients had to be pureed with fruit in a blender and fed to him through a large syringe, one end of which was attached to a rubber bulb.

His blood pressure was high, and he had extremely poor peripheral circulation. His lower legs, feet, hands, face, nose and ears were cold to the touch.

The patient was placed in a private hospital. He was treated for five weeks. And at the end of that time he could walk, talk and conduct a conversation at will. His physician, unknown to me, had recorded his attempts at conversation daily. Gradually discernible speech emerged from formerly unintelligible mumbling. The tape was startling to hear.

PARALYSIS OF LONG DURATION

The stroke patient with long-term established paralysis will respond nicely to EDTA chelation therapy. The first case of this type treated is still clear in my mind because at that time I had never treated a stroke that had been established for more than two years. We had been told as students, many years before, that if progress is not seen by that time, none would be forthcoming. Without attempting to test this theory, I simply took it on faith, and never accepted a paralyzed case that was more than two years post-stroke.

About fifteen years ago a young lady brought her father to us for treatment. He had suffered a stroke seven years previously, and could barely sit in his wheelchair. His head hung to the left, his mouth was open. Saliva drooled from his extended tongue. His right arm was enclosed in a sling, and the hand was cold to the touch. His right leg occupied a lucite cast which extended from the foot to the knee. A canvas strap had been fastened about his waist to keep him from falling out of the wheelchair. He could not walk, eat or care for himself in any way; he was totally dependent.

"I want you to treat my father," she said.

"I don't think I can help him," I said. "His stroke is too well established after all this time."

"Doctor, I'm a nurse at St. Mary's Hospital here in town, and I can care for him. I will do anything you want done."

"But Miss, I don't think the treatment will work. I don't want to promise something I can't deliver. You would be wasting your money."

"It's my money, and I want to spend it on my dad, whether it helps him or not. I have seen several of the stroke patients you have treated and they all do remarkably well. I know chelation can't hurt him. I insist you treat him. I want him to have the chance of getting well."

I shall never be able to thank that lady enough. She rekindled my desire to help abandoned chronic disease cases. It is an effort sometimes to question the established methods of treatment. It requires a flexible mind, and just when my thinking gets a little starchy, I remember this lady and her dad.

This sixty-eight year old gentleman required twenty-eight treatments before his blood chemistries and arterial tracings returned to normal and remained stable. Little by little he came out of his bodily prison. He gradually began to say a few clear words, sleep soundly and, according to his daughter, maintain a more cheerful demeanor.

Soon he was able to walk with a four-legged aluminum walking device. He progressed to crutches. Aerobic exercises were prescribed at this point, and the patient determinedly pursued them. In a short time he had graduated to two canes, then one cane. Finally, he could walk without assistance, care for himself, talk and do all the other things a normal person might do.

He left one day to join his wife in a small town outside Kansas City, and they have been self-sufficient ever since.

At his insistence, we kept one of his canes, as a pointed reminder of his case. He said he wants me to remember that I didn't want to treat him at the beginning.

For the past fifteen years or so, stroke patients have been treated with EDTA at our clinic. There are hundreds of stroke case histories in our files with equally good results. In the near future we will be publishing these findings in the medical literature.

10

Chelation Therapy
And Senility

Nearly everyone recognizes senility, a condition that is seen throughout the world. A small child recognizes that grandpa is no longer capable of conducting his personal affairs in a normal manner. He may have trouble remembering things, and he may have difficulty speaking and thinking coherently. Typically the senile patient will have lost the ability to complete a sentence. The attention span is short, and the mind wanders.

Commonly the senile patient is an elderly man or woman who has gradually evolved into a senile mental state with advancing age. It is a rare patient who is merely senile. Usually patients have several other afflictions. Occlusive vascular disease, diabetes, heart disease and arthritis are commonly seen in senile patients. The patient may have a generalized functional loss of his special senses. He may not hear, smell things or taste things as he formerly could. Joints and muscles are stiff and reflexes are slow.

On the other hand, the patient may appear to be perfectly healthy. His mental capacity may be very poor, however.

Nora, a fifty-four year old female, appeared slim and healthy when she arrived at McDonagh Medical Center several years ago. She could walk briskly and used her arms and legs in a normal fashion. She did not appear to be in distress.

"Nora, I'm Dr. McDonagh. How are you today?"

"Fine."

"Have you been having any difficulties?"

"No, I'm fine."

"Well then, why have you come to see me today?"

"My husband brought me."

"Can you tell me your full name?"

"I'm Nora."

"Tell me what you did last evening."

"I'm Nora. I got up yesterday and we...I'm Nora."

"Nora, what did you have for breakfast this morning?"

"I'm Nora. I had some...I'm fine."

This is a typical conversation with a patient suffering from senility. This lady's case was quite dramatic because she was severely impaired at a relatively young age. It is interesting and curious that senility and vascular degenerative disease is occurring in many people at an earlier age than would be expected.

Senility can result as a secondary consequence of many disease processes. Several factors may be operating. Toxic chemical products, resulting in an infectious disease, commonly cause mental aberrations. Disturbances in the brain chemistry from lack of enzyme activity, malabsorption or lack of vitamins or minerals, or faulty brain glucose metabolism can contribute to the development of senility. The most commonly caused cases of senility are the result of vascular occlusion in the arteries which feed blood to the brain.

An article appearing in *Medical Tribune,* on November 25, 1981 verifies the chief cause of senility as circulatory lack. Dr. Louis Sokoloff was awarded the 1981 Albert Lasker Clinical Medical Research Award for developing a new method to measure the brain's metabolic activity, an accomplishment with promising diagnostic and therapeutic implications. Dr. Sokoloff has been termed a "scientist's scientist" by his colleagues, and it has been said that he should receive the Nobel prize for his work.

At the National Institute of Mental Health, which he joined in 1953, Dr. Sokoloff led a team in making the first major study of cerebral blood flow in the normal aging brain. They established that brain blood flow and oxygen consumption do not change with age in normal individuals. With this study, Sokoloff and his colleagues refuted the prior notion that aging is associated with necessary and programmed deterioration of brain function, blood flow and metabolism. They thereby showed that one cause of deterioration of the central nervous system is not the consequence of chronological aging, but of arteriosclerosis and a secondary reduction in cerebral metabolic rate of primary organic brain disease.

The great majority of chelated senility patients will awaken from their mental confusion gradually as they progress through the treatment. Some of them, however, go through the process, treatment after treatment with no apparent benefit. Then, after several treatments, they seem suddenly to regain normal mentation. It is as dramatic as snapping your fingers, or turning on a light in a dark room.

Jim K.'s case was a good example.

"It is good to see you again, Jim."

"Well, doctor, it has been almost a year since I finished my treatment and I have really come to see you and show you how well I'm doing."

"You certainly look wonderful."

"I feel just great, Doctor. You know, I want to thank you and your wonderful staff for helping me. I must have been quite difficult to care for."

"We've had worse, Jim. The important thing now is that you are feeling so good and living a normal life again."

"Well, I want to tell you some of the changes that have happened in the past year. Now that I can drive again, I got the old car out of the garage and traded it off on a new one. I have a whole new wardrobe, and I'm starting my own business."

"How many treatment infusions did you take before you realized you were making good progess? You know, when you first began treatment, you were out of it mentally. You didn't know who you were, or where you were."

"Well, Doc, I dimly recall you saying one day that I just finished my seventeenth treatment. You were asking how I felt. To tell the truth, I never knew I had the previous sixteen."

This gentleman, now seventy-three, was sixty-eight years old at the time of his first treatment. He could not walk without assistance from his wife. They lived on a large corner lot which had a considerable amount of flowers and shrubbery. Prior to the onset of treatment, the wife had put the house up for sale because the upkeep was too much for her, and he could not help out.

The patient had a body and fender repair business that he was forced to sell to his brother-in-law due to advancing arteriosclerosis and senility. For several years he was unable to care for himself, feed himself, or do any of the usual work around the house. He was severely withdrawn and depressed.

When he first came to see us as a patient, he was depressed to the point of suicide. While under treatment, he would ask his wife to divorce him so she might find another man, and live a relatively normal life. A pitiful situation, indeed.

This gentleman has salvaged his life, and that of his wife. He has an entirely new printing business, one that he was able to devise and operate himself. It has been a privilege and a delight to have been able to aid him, a wonderfully fulfilling feeling.

To say that life is precious is not to invite challenge. However the quality of life must be top-notch to make it precious. The usual medical treatment of patients with senility is shallow and incomplete. A high percentage of senility cases eventually have a stroke, which is frequently terminal, or they suffer severe incapacitation.

A visit to any nursing home will confirm this. You will note that virtually all of the nursing home patients suffer from senility and/or the aftermath of occlusive artery disease to the brain, chiefly stroke and its sequellae. In the dining area

Chelation Therapy And Senility 69

you will be impressed with the brilliance and glitter that is reflected from a vast array of wheelchairs. They are lined up, wheel to wheel, along the dining table like bicycles in a sporting goods store.

In America we warehouse our old people. They are perceived as an undesirable and unproductive segment of the population. They need large amounts of money from the Social Security administration for their subsistence. They require large amounts of health care every year. In their senescence they burden their children and hold back the growing family economically.

What would happen if we could change all this, if senility could be prevented and its economic impact removed?

Basic to the human psyche is the need to contribute, to work gainfully. No one really wants to sit on the sidelines of life and be dependent on others. There are legions of Colonel Sanders types that could have a very positive influence on our economy, and indeed, our political system, if they could achieve and maintain physical and mental function.

How many promising and innovative sculptors, painters or businessmen would make their contribution to society if there were enough physicans practicing chelation therapy and removing the stigma and burden of senility?

We tend to take people for granted, especially those we love the most. If you have a loved one who is developing senility, or if you yourself have noticed slippage in your mental capacity, I urge you to investigate the chelation treatment concept. Ideally, of course, it is much easier to prevent the onslaught of senility by detecting and treating the condition in its earlier stages.

There can be no more loving gesture from a son or daughter than that of giving their parents or in-laws the ability to live their lives in a clear mental state.

Medicine, as it is currently practiced in the United States, cannot offer this advantage. I feel that what physicians do, they do well. They just cannot go far enough. I believe that all "schools of thought" can share or blend their experience and attain superb results routinely.

Most physicans practice excellent medicine, and do the very best that they can do for their patients. But it seems that an informed public must assert itself and ask doctors to investigate EDTA chelation therapy for themselves.

Treatment takes time, and is not a hospital procedure. It requires a bit of insight into multiple diagnostic problems. However, it is not that difficult to learn, and results are more than worth the effort. It is no longer necessary for an elderly person to vegetate on life's sidelines. The elderly patient has the feeling, knowledge and experience that took a lifetime to accumulate. He wants to share it with his loved ones and his country. It is up to others to act in his behalf.

11
Chelation Therapy And Peripheral Vascular Disease

The legs are commonly involved with peripheral vascular disease, also males are affected more than premenopausal females.

A common symptom is intermittent claudication (intermittent limping) cramping pain, numbness, tightness or severe fatigue in the muscle group being exercised. The patient must stop all activity, rest a moment or two, and the pain promptly disappears. Commonly, the calf muscles of the legs are involved, but muscles of the low back, buttocks, thigh and foot may also be affected.

Absent or diminished pulses are found distal to the obstruction. Signs of ischemia are present distally, also. The extremity is cold when compared to the limb of the opposite side.

Severe coldness, even in warm weather is a sign of advanced arterial disease. I have seen patients who wore long underwear, socks or gloves to bed throughout the summer months.

Skin color distal to the obstruction is usually abnormal. Grayish or reddish color is not unusual. The skin becomes dry, shiny and tight. There is absence of hair on the skin distal to the obstruction.

Much like the root of a plant or tree, an artery has many branches. The flow of blood must be widely distributed to nourish all tissue cells. Each series of branches is smaller than the trunk vessel from which they arose, and the farther the parent artery wanders from the heart, the smaller and more narrow it becomes.

It would be reasonable to think, therefore, that at the periphery these hair-like vessels might be the victims of occlusion more often than the larger main arterial channels. This might be so, except for the fact that the most distant vessels—those of the hands, arms, feet and legs—have their circulation assisted by the motion of the limbs. Muscular activity is necessary to allow the limbs to move, and this same activity helps circulate the blood. The constant give and take of gentle muscular squeezing gives the smaller vessels additional pumping assistance, keeping circulation at the periphery efficient and preventing early occlusion.

Disease of these vessels is not as common because of physical activity. When people slow down due to advancing age, or because of disease, or because of poor health habits, problems in these vessels begin to surface.

Of all the chronic diseases, diabetes is perhaps the most common cause of leg ulcers, swelling, discoloration and gangrene. More legs and feet and toes have been amputated due to diabetes-caused gangrene than for any other cause.

Other causes of peripheral vascular disease include viral or bacterial infections of the arteriole wall, or the nerve supply to the arteriole, with subsequent occlusion, ulceration, infection or gangrene.

Sustained pressure on a body part, or muscular area can cause loss of circulation. Tiny arterioles are compressed, and no nutrient-laden blood can pass. Cells become dormant as toxic wastes build up and nutrients are denied. Eventually a segment of tissue dies. It rots, sloughs, and an ulcer is born. Bed sores are a familiar example.

Because of atherosclerosis the circulation was poor to

start with, and healing of the ulcer now will be difficult. Secondary infection is the rule rather than the exception.

Inherited hypersensitivity to tobacco causes some people to develop spasms and loss of blood supply to the fingers, toes, hands and feet. The disease is called Berger's disease.

These patients commonly are addicted to cigarette smoking. Unless the patient gives up tobacco, treatment is ineffective and eventually gangrene of the extremities develops.

Surgeons have told me the first request many of these patients make when awakening after amputation surgery is for a cigarette. How very sad it is, because as the patient continues to smoke, the problem continues, and an additional amputation will be required.

I shall always remember the case history of a man I met in Topeka, Kansas one evening. About two years ago, Dr. Charles Rudolph and I were invited to address a group of people living in a retirement community.

Arriving early, we met and talked with several members of the audience. One man, about fifty years old, was sitting in a wheelchair. He had Berger's disease. Multiple amputations had taken both legs, his left arm and several fingers of his right hand. Holding a cigarette in the surgically deformed right hand, he admitted to being a chain smoker.

"I had all of my amputations at V.A. hospitals, and because I'm a veteran, it didn't cost me anything," he said.

"Well, that's something at least," I said.

"You know they really take good care of the patients. They have all sorts of people visiting you and giving you gifts."

"You mean volunteer groups giving you candy and stuff like that?"

"Yeah. And cigarettes. At least three different groups come once a week. They each give me a carton of cigarettes. When I get ready to leave, my dresser drawer is full to the top with packages of cigarettes."

"Didn't your doctor tell you to quit smoking?" I asked.

"Yes, but he had a cigarette in his hand at the time."

Giving cigarettes to this man was about as sensible as

firemen squirting gasoline on a blaze to put it out.

Another peripheral vascular disease condition is Raynaud's disease. It is usually seen in women. The arteries in the hands and fingers are affected. The hand becomes blanched, painful and cold. It is temporarily relieved by placing the hand in warm water.

When occlusive disease of a major artery occurs, it is the downstream tissue, now cut off from its blood supply, that suffers. Typically, occlusion progresses until gangrene rears its ugly head. If, for example, occlusion occurs in the iliac arteries of the thigh, or the femoral-popliteal area behind the knee, it is the foot that becomes discolored, swollen, painful, and eventually infected. It cannot function. By the time gangrene develops, the occlusive process has worsened and amputation is the usual treatment. The patient is commonly told that nothing else can be done to save his life, for the gangrene will kill him eventually.

The pain of gangrene is excruciating. It does not take much convincing for the patient to submit to surgery. I have had patients with gangrene say they want their leg removed if it will stop the pain.

It does not have to be that way. Even with gangrene present, EDTA treatment can prevent amputation and reverse the disease condition in most cases. Two examples are the following cases.

Mrs. Jean Alberti, a lady in her late forties, was told by several doctors in Peoria, Illinois that she had advanced occlusive disease of both legs. The left foot was badly swollen and had turned maroon in color when she was first seen at our clinic. There was a black spot on her heel and the entire great toe was black. She could not tolerate pressure on the foot, not even that of a bedsheet. She walked poorly with the aid of crutches. Her usual facial expression was that of a person in pain.

Vascular testing confirmed severe arterial occlusive disease of both legs. She also showed poor kidney and heart function, and abnormally elevated cholesterol, triglycerides, uric acid and blood sugar.

Infusion treatments with EDTA were begun. She was also given the usual supplementary support, diet modification, exercise therapy and other ancillary help. For example, during the early portion of her treatment she required narcotics for pain and sleeping pills at night.

After a few treatments the body's healing ability began to assert itself. She noticed reduced pain, and the ability to get about easier. This was followed by increased energy, loss of fatigue, and reduced need for pain medication. She stopped taking her sleeping pills after two weeks.

The nail of the great toe was removed. It had been harboring an infection underneath. She could now limp about by herself, using a cane. She became cheerful and jolly.

Following the inactive phase of her treatment she had no problem with her legs, feet, toes, heart, or anything else for that matter. She evolved into an enthusiastic live-wire and dispensed positivity wherever she went.

I'm happy for her, and I'm happy I was able to help. Before starting treatment her husband told me the doctors in Peoria advised immediate amputation of the right leg below the knee. They told him the left leg would have to come off three to six months later.

Another case that would have resulted in amputation had it not been for EDTA is that of Mr. Edward Creamer. This patient, age sixty-four, had been suffering from the gradual development of a napkin-ring-type of occlusion in the lower aorta, the largest artery in the body.

In 1979, Mr. Creamer consulted Dr. Denton Cooley in Houston, Texas. Arteriogram tests diagnosed the problem and Dr. Cooley operated. A portion of the aorta containing the ring of occlusive slag was removed. A tubular graft of synthetic cloth was stitched into place.

Mr. Creamer had no more difficulty for a year or so. Thereafter, he began to notice weakness in his legs. He ignored it as long as he could. Gradually, however, weakness became fatigue. Pain was finally added to the equation. His feet had turned a dark grey-maroon color and were constantly swollen and painful.

In 1982 when he could no longer walk one block without severe incapacitating pain in his legs, he returned to Houston.

Dr. Cooley again performed arteriography. The test showed advanced occlusive disease in both legs and feet. Mr. Creamer states Dr. Cooley told him he needed to amputate one foot immediately, and the other one in six months.

"Isn't there something that can be done to save my feet?" Mr. Creamer asked.

"No, nothing can be done except surgical amputation. I'll make the arrangements."

The patient, after some thought, checked himself out of the hospital. Shortly after that he became a chelation patient. After nine treatments the pain greatly diminished and his feet returned to normal color. He could walk six blocks without pain.

After twenty-six treatments he resumed his normal lifestyle.

Gangrene does not have to mean the loss of the limb as was formerly thought. It is the end result of vascular occlusive disease, and must be treated as such. "Watchful expectancy" is detrimental to the survival of the limb. Aggressive, early treatment is a must. Vascular occlusive disease from whatever cause, is favorably reversed by the chelation concept which incorporates nutrient supplementation, dietary improvement, exercise of an aerobic nature done daily, and of course, EDTA.

No longer is a patient forced to choose between the loss of his leg, or the loss of his life by the gangrene. The human body has the remarkable ability to heal itself. With this treatment procedure, the relentless disease process is held at bay. The ammunition needed to conduct this victorious battle is supplied in adequate amounts, but the body's healing power is the fighter, the doer. Perhaps because chelation attacks all areas of abnormality simultaneously, the body can retrench and concentrate its ability to fight. Without this approach, the body's defenses are spread thinly about, ineffectively fighting on many fronts at once.

One thing is known. Gangrene is no threat today once chelation treatment is started. In our files there are more than twenty years' experience proving this.

12
Chelation Therapy and Diabetes

Diabetes and its counterpart, hypoglycemia, are diseases characterized by disturbances in the delicate balance of the body's sugar chemistry. The sugar, glucose, is a normal blood constituent used as a source of energy. Insulin and some twenty enzymatic chemical reactions are necessary to utilize this energy. The efficiency of insulin is influenced by ascorbic acid (vitamin C).

For normal functioning of the human body, concentration of glucose in the blood must be maintained within narrow limits. The normal range is 65 to 120 milligram percent. It is insulin that regulates this level within the normal range. Insulin is produced by cell clusters in the pancreas called the islets of Langerhans. From here, insulin enters the blood.

The amount of glucose in the blood will vary, depending on what the patient eats, and on how much he eats. Insulin must be metered by the pancreas in just the right amounts to deal with the intake. Too little circulating insulin permits the blood sugar level to rise abnormally—the so-called diabetic effect. Too much insulin in the blood is equally bad because it produces the hypoglycemic state. There are probably as many people suffering from hypoglycemia as from diabetes.

Normally, when the body has more sugar than it requires, the excess is stored in the liver as glycogen. It remains there until it is required by the body as energy fuel. In the diabetic, too much circulating glucose causes trouble.

Diabetes is a total vasculitis. It affects every blood vessel in the body. In a diabetic patient, the basement membrane and the endothelial layer comprising the innermost cells that line the interior of the blood vessels are abnormal. There is an accumulation in these cells of insoluble, amorphous material called "ground substance" because of its appearance under the microscope. It stains homogeneously, giving the appearance of ground glass.

If we were to look at a tiny hair-like arteriole under the electron microscope, the tubular structure would have the appearance of chicken-wire fencing material. The cells that make up the arteriole have numerous gaps and spaces between them.

Under normal conditions, nutrients such as vitamins, minerals, proteins, hormones, enzymes, fats, carbohydrates and so on, all are able to ooze through these openings to nourish tissue cells. Cellular wastes are able to enter the capillary vessel in the same manner.

In a diabetic patient, the *ground substance* plugs the pores in the vessel wall. The basement membrane thickens, and the tiniest of vessels are no longer able to function properly, making it impossible for nutrients to ooze through blood vessel walls normally.

The endocrine system, and all other tissues of the diabetic, are perpetually on the dangerous edge of malnourishment and oxygen starvation. It is thought that the abnormal amounts of circulating blood sugar are responsible for the chemical and enzymatic changes that cause the basement membrane to thicken. The same mechanism is probably responsible for the thickening and roughening that occurs all over the vascular system. Atherosclerosis is off to a running start early in the diabetic patient.

Diabetes is a defect in the metabolism of carbohydrates. It is the third largest cause of death in the United States, exceeded only by cardiovascular disease and cancer. It is the leading cause of blindness.

Patients with diabetes must be careful with any infection that may be contracted. Healing is slow, and immunity is usually poor. These patients have a greater incidence of heart disease. Arthritis and gangrene are frequently found. Accordingly, the risk for these diseases is multiplied many times.

A broken bone, influenza, pneumonia, kidney or bladder infection, prostate or pelvic infections, skin infections, or a simple trimming of the toenails must be managed with care and diligence.

The retinal membranes of the eyes suffer tremendous damage from diabetes. Cataracts, hemorrhages, retinitis, macular degeneration and early blindness are not unusual.

Truly this is a vascular occlusive disease which has run amok in our affluent society. It causes damage to many organ systems simultaneously, and in so doing, it causes a dreadful suppression on the body's ability to resist disease.

When there is persistently elevated blood sugar, diabetes is diagnosed. If one of your parents or grandparents had dia-betes, the chances are good that you are carrying the gene for the development of diabetes. This does not mean that you will develop the disease, for there is much that can be done to keep it at bay. If both of your parents had frank diabetes, you have, or most likely will have the problem.

A call to the American Diabetic Association of Arizona, during a recent visit to Scottsdale, resulted in the following information:

There are approximately six million diabetics in the U.S.A. The figure cannot be verified, because the ADA believes at least half of these are "in the closet," as the society represen-tative told me. Many people either have not been diagnosed yet, or they don't want others to know. Considering the ear-ly, wholesale ravaging of the circulatory system by this disease, this attitude is destructive to the patient. In Arizona, there are an estimated 100,000 diabetics, and a new case develops at the rate of one per hour.

The ADA's mission is to educate the public about the disease, because diabetes is not terribly difficult to manage. Using some preventive approaches, chelation with EDTA, dietary modification, exercise programs and increased dietary fiber intake, diabetes can be reversed and held in check indefinitely.

In about 50% of cases, diabetes is inherited. It has been estimated that more than one out of five persons in this country carries a recessive gene for the disease.

In 1934, C.G. King and co-workers at the University of Pittsburgh showed that guinea pigs maintained on low levels of ascorbic acid developed degeneration of the islets of Langerhans. Could low levels of vitamin C predispose patients to diabetes? If so, is there a role for vitamin C in the treatment of the disease?

Banerjee, starting in 1943, showed the disturbed carbohydrate metabolism as seen in scurvy is due to a deficiency of insulin secretion and a chronic deficiency of vitamin C, which may be one of the etiological factors of diabetes mellitis in human subjects. In 1958 he published additional studies confirming his earlier work. His 1964 paper contained the very suggestive results of the work in the intestinal absorption of glucose. It was found that the intestinal absorption of sugar was about doubled when animals were deprived of ascorbic acid. This function returned to normal when test animals received ascorbic acid.

Applied to human beings, this observation would mean that the intestines of diabetics, who may exist on chronic, low levels of ascorbic acid, permit a much more rapid absorption of glucose to higher levels, and put abnormal stress on the already strained insulin production in their pancreas.

The intimate relationship between insulin and ascorbic acid has been noted numerous times. When insulin is injected, there is a fall in the ascorbic acid levels of blood serum in man, dogs, and rats, as shown by Ralli and Sherry in 1940 and 1948. Haid, in 1941, also noted this drop, not only after insulin injection, but in patients in insulin shock (hypoglycemic shock). Previously, in 1939, Wille reported that ascorbic acid is helpful to schizophrenics receiving insulin shock treatments. This scientist also produced evidence that ascorbic acid acts to raise the blood sugar levels in hypoglycemic attacks. She showed that prolonged administration of ascorbic acid will prevent these low blood sugar attacks.

Ascorbic acid potentiates the action of insulin and therefore makes it possible to derive the same effect with much less insulin. This was observed in 1939 by Bartelheimer and was accidently confirmed by Rogoff and co-workers in 1944. Pfleger and Scholl noted that ascorbic acid so improved the action of insulin that a diabetic could control sugar tolerance with a lower level of insulin.

The combination of ascorbic acid with the oral medications used to treat diabetes is helpful in avoiding some of the undesirable vascular effects of diabetic treatments.

For the past twenty years we have noted the benefical effects of high doses of ascorbic acid on the diabetic condition. Hundreds of patients have had unusually speedy improvement, even those advanced cases with multiple diagnostic problems in addition to diabetes. Diabetes may be prevented by the long-term ingestion of daily optimal amounts of ascorbic acid.

HOW WE TREAT DIABETES TODAY

At least 80% of the adult diabetics living in the United States are or were obese. In the diabetic male an increase in weight above the accepted normal is associated with a considerable increase in the risk of dying. For example, an individual 20% above his accepted normal weight has a 350% greater mortality risk. Weight reduction for the obese diabetic, therefore, is a must.

Figures from Nutrition Research Laboratories, Department of Preventive Medicine, Washington University School of Medicine, reveal that the prevalence of diabetes is increasing in the United States at a more rapid rate than the growth of the total population. According to current death rates studies by the World Health Organization, the United

States is one of the leaders in diabetic deaths among the economically developed countries. Diabetes is closely associated with many other chronic degenerative diseases.

Chronic disease prevention and reversal, therefore, must hinge on resolving the diabetic problem. Normalization of improper carbohydrate metabolism is of prime importance. The addition of large doses of ascorbic acid to the EDTA infusion as well as adequate supplementation by mouth, enables the patient to turn the corner toward health quickly and easily.

An aerobic exercise program performed for twenty minutes daily can drop elevated blood sugar forty to fifty points within six weeks, with no other change in the diabetic's lifestyle. Diabetics can increase their tolerance for sugar and decrease their dependence on insulin by engaging in moderate exercise after meals, according to an article in the *New England Journal of Medicine,* April 17, 1980.

The wise patient will want to change other habits toward those more healthy. Reduction of dietary fat, sugar and alcohol is sensible. Smoking, because of its effect on the circulation of blood, should be stopped. Plethysmographic tracings of digital arteries (fingers) in our files show time and again the constrictive effect of smoking. Substances in the inhaled cigarette smoke, probably nicotine, cause the arteries to become spastic, and blood flow to be drastically reduced.

One patient had not smoked for three hours and digital tracings were made. She was then allowed to smoke for ten minutes. Again, tracings of the arteries in her fingers were made. The tests taken after smoking showed a reduction of blood flow by 400%. No diabetic can afford to smoke.

In addition to vitamin C, B complex vitamins, trace minerals, vitamin E and inositol are added to the diabetic supplement program, to quicken the reversal of metabolic imbalance. Beta carotene is given in multiple daily oral doses. This precursor of vitamin A is necessary to aid the recovery of basement membranes of blood vessels, cell membranes, skin and all other mucous membranes in the body.

Diabetic patients respond exceptionally well to EDTA chelation therapy probably because so much pathology resides in blood vessel membranes.

SOME CASES OF INTEREST

About ten years ago an elderly man requested consultation about his wife. It seemed she was having constant nausea and vomiting. This had persisted for two weeks. He stated she could not get out of bed. She was light-headed, and would faint after taking three or four steps. If she attempted to eat, invariably the food was vomited. She complained of severe pain in the low back, and had difficulty urinating. Her temperature had been over 100 F. for a week.

"She's also dried out, Doc. Her skin is sure looking dry. You know she was a diabetic a few years back. She has been taking medicine from a doctor, but she didn't like the way it made her feel, so she stopped taking it a few months back. Do you think I should bring her to the office?"

"No, no," I said. "Take her directly to the hospital. I will make arrangements immediately."

When this lady was examined in the hospital she was indeed diabetic. Her blood sugar was more than 1000 milligrams percent. She was semi-comatose and could not talk or answer questions clearly. Her mind wandered.

On the heel of her right foot was a black gangrenous area about the size of a silver dollar. A similar-sized area was located on the top surface of the other foot. Her teeth were in poor repair and one central incisor tooth projected outward to press against her lip. In this area, apparently where the tooth had been rubbing, was a circular area of gangrene approximately the size of a green pea. It was coal-black in color, however it was not draining freely. The gangrenous areas on her feet were draining a yellowish fluid.

There was an active infection in her kidneys and urinary bladder. On the surface of the right lower abdomen was a large ballooning hernia. She had this for some time, however it had enlarged by the strain on the abdominal muscles caused by retching and vomiting. Her skin, hair and nails were a disaster. Her toenails had turned black on both feet, and were misshapen and twisted. Her fingernails showed the same problem, but were not in as advanced a state of degeneration. Her hair was snow white and exceptionally sparse. One could see the entire scalp.

Her skin, especially, was in very poor condition. It was dehydrated, with many folds of loose hanging skin over the hands, arms, legs and hips. One could pick up loose folds of skin three to four inches long by two inches deep. It appeared dark grey in color, and had deep cracks and fissures in many locations.

During the hospital stay the infection was treated with antibiotics. Treatment with insulin, intravenous fluids, dietary manipulation, and eventually surgical correction of the hernia, was done. After her discharge from the hospital, the patient was started on daily infusions of EDTA. The gangrene, which had stabilized, and for the most part had stopped draining pus, had not changed color. It was black in all three areas.

As a result of the chelation treatment, gradually her skin color improved, as did the skin turgor. The gangrene cleared. Her hair began to change color and grow. Eventually she regained a full head of thick dark brown hair.

By the time she was released from active treatment, her strength and stamina had increased. She could walk two miles briskly every day. She looked and felt better than she had in twenty years, according to her husband.

Another case that should be mentioned is the case of Mr. S.M. This tall asthenic man, age sixty-eight, was buying a pair of shoes a few doors down the street when the shoe salesman noted a red streak on one leg, extending from the foot to the mid-calf. The patient was a long-standing diabetic. He had been gradually losing vision, as well as his sense of pain and pressure in his feet. He stepped on a nail protruding from a board, but did not feel it. A day or two later, the shoe salesman noticed the infection. The patient did not see well enough to recognize it, and he couldn't feel pain due to his advanced diabetic neuropathy (nerve damage). He was guided by his wife when he entered the office. She said he was legally blind, and could see only blurred images four or five feet away.

He was examined and tested. Diabetes, congestive heart failure, hypertension and severe peripheral vascular disease were present. There was a puncture wound on the bottom of one foot, and it oozed pus. A red streak had indeed developed and extended half way up the lower leg.

He had been told by his opthalmologist that his eyes were beyond help. The tiny arterioles of the retinal membranes had become arteriosclerotic, brittle and leaky. Serum exudates oozed from the damaged blood vessels and congealed onto the retinal membrane itself, causing loss of vision. This is not uncommon in diabetics. As the diabetic effect on the body accelerates, more insulin is required to combat blood sugar elevations, and to counter increased fatigue. Visual deterioration continues and more visual capacity is lost.

In the early stages opthamologists can attempt to *vulcanize* or cauterize the tiny leaking vessels with minute pinpoints of heat generated by a laser beam of concentrated, focused light. The vessel is closed off just above the area that is leaking. Scar tissue will form and circulation will not proceed past that point. Temporarily, the procedure is effective. No more leaking occurs from those cauterized vessels. No more loss of retinal "seeing" ability occurs because no more fluid can escape the cauterized vessel.

The procedure is temporary, unfortunately, because all vessels in the eye (and body in general) will continue to deteriorate. That is what diabetes is all about. Laser photocoagulation does nothing to combat diabetes, or atherosclerosis in the eye's vessels.

Other vessels in the retina will begin to leak later, and the loss of vision continues. In this patient's case, high blood pressure pushed the problem along. One day, a point of no return is reached. The opthalmologist cannot continue to obliterate arteries, or too little retinal blood supply will remain. Excessive loss of blood supply will destroy the retina, the way a stroke destroys brain tissue. Eventually so much retinal area has been damaged by hemorrhages, serum protein, cholesterol and fat that blindness results.

Mr. M's opthalmologist had told him he was going to be totally blind in a few months, and nothing could be done to prevent it.

Could something be done?

Treatment was begun. Slowly, progress was seen. His insulin was able to be reduced from 70 units per day to 60, then 50. His blood pressure and heart function improved. The patient was started on an aerobic exercise program. He pedaled a stationary bicycle non-stop for twenty minutes, then forty-five, and then one hour. To keep his mind off the exercise procedure, the patient did his workouts in front of the TV, watching his favorite programs.

Insulin requirements continued to drop. Large doses of B complex and vitamin C were given four times daily. He was advised to increase his fiber intake by eating three cooked vegetables at each meal, including breakfast. Whole grain cereals and bread were advised, but refined carbohydrates were restricted.

He continued to make progress, gaining strength daily. The effect of EDTA on his eyes was exciting:

"Doc, I can now see across the room!" he said. Later he exclaimed: "Doc, I can see clear to the end of the block!"

After completing the fortieth treatment, he returned to a full and active retirement life. He began to drive his car again. He worked in his garden and assisted his wife with the housework. He now required only four units of insulin daily. Re-examination by his opthalmologist was exciting for everyone, patient, wife and doctor.

The opthalmologist stated with amazement: "I don't know what has caused this, but now we can do something to help. There are only a few tiny leaks at this stage. The rest of them have healed and the retina has cleared. I'm going to put you into the hospital for laser coagulation."

Three months following the procedure, the patient had stabilized his visual acuity at 20/30, a remarkable comeback from blindness. A short time later, I received a call from the opthalmologist.

"I wanted to discuss our patient, Mr. S.M.," he said.

"I'll be glad to help, if I can," I said.

"The patient tried to tell me you used some type of fluid dripped into his veins."

"That's correct."

"He said it was composed of vitamins and other things that cleaned out the arteries. Just what is the active ingredient in the solution, doctor?"

"Just vitamins and EDTA," I answered.

"You must be keeping something from me," he said incredulously. "We all know that won't work!"

"It does work, and it works well, doctor. Come over for a visit. We can pull charts. You can see the results for yourself. When would you like to come?"

"I'll have to call you later."

Unfortunately, he never did come to see for himself. He could not use the treatment for his patients anyhow, probably, without bringing down the wrath of his collegues.

For our patients, we strive to obtain the very best results possible. Our primary allegiance is to the patients. All other considerations are secondary.

Physicians interested in the elimination of disabling diseases such as arthritis, heart disease, diabetes, vascular disease and so forth, have found through long experience that there are several common threads that weave themselves through all chronic debilitating conditions. Blood supply and proper nutrition are the most important of these, and they are inseparable, if one hopes to prevent, stop or reverse disability and dysfunction. One of the problems is to determine just what each patient requires to balance his metabolic chemistry. A tailored program, made to fit each patient's unique requirements, is necessary. No two patients have the same chemical balance or deficiencies. Periodic re-examination is advised to *fine tune* and adjust dosages of nutrients.

At McDonagh Medical Center, part of the patient testing program includes a questionnaire that asks the patient about his past and present health status. Past problems, mild, moderate or severe are important.

A dietary survey is part of the questionnaire. Patients are asked to list the foods they eat, and the number of times per week they eat them. The patient simply places a check mark at the appropriate place on the form.

Information gathered in this manner is fed into a computer. The print-out will reveal the patient's obvious problems as well as the subtle ones. It will also predict illness that has not yet surfaced. Vitamin imbalance is determined with relative accuracy. These findings alert the physician to areas that need further testing and study, allowing him to *zero in* quickly to problem areas.

The computer will provide a list of vitamins, glandular extracts, enzymes and other nutrients that are necessary to correct imbalances. The dosage and time of day each nutrient is to be taken is stated.

Large doses of intravenous vitamins, especially ascorbic acid (vitamin C) is a great help in the majority of patients. The indications for large doses of this vitamin are too numerous to mention, but some of our reasons follow. An excellent and interesting book for the nonprofessional reader is Irwin Stone's book, *The Healing Factor*. This book covers the benefits of megadoses of C to virtually every system of the body.

Ascorbic acid is added to every intravenous solution, with very few exceptions. It has been found by R.R. Becker and his team that ascorbic acid deprivation greatly increased cholesterol synthesis. The greater the deprivation of ascorbic acid, the more cholesterol accumulated in the tissues. Coronary atherosclerosis (plugging of the coronary artery) appears to be in part, a possible result of insufficient ingestion of ascorbic acid.

Increased intake of ascorbic acid brings down cholesterol levels in human beings.

13
Will Modern Medicine
Let You Live?
The Medical Literature of
EDTA Chelation Therapy

In the booklet, *Reversing Degeneration and Aging Through Chelation,* the following appears inside the front cover:

"The scientific literature dealing with EDTA, which was first synthesized by German chemists of I.G. Farbenindustrie about 1937, has achieved relatively vast proportions.

"EDTA holds a singular position in the world of coordination chemistry. Among analytical chemists EDTA has an ideal structure as a chelation ligand because of the frequent occurrence among divalent and trivalent metallic ions of the coordination number 6. As a superior chelating agent it is surpassed only by a single compound, namely the trans-1, 2-diaminocyclohexanetetracetic acid. Nevertheless, EDTA is probably the most popular of chelating agents among analytical chemists because of its availability and because chemical activity can be accurately and mathematically predicted.

"Because of the widespread use of EDTA in industry, chemical laboratories, food and biological preservation, the scientific chemical literature on EDTA now numbers in the thousands of papers. A large body of this literature has been discussed by F.J. Welcher (1961), *The Analytical Uses of Ethylenediamine Tetraacetic Acid,* D. vann Nostrand, Princeton, 336 pages.

"Clinical research on the medical applications of EDTA in atherosclerosis, and cardiovascular diseases, cardiac arrhythmias and digitalis intoxication, heavy metal poisoning, sclerotic diseases, calcinosis and hypercalcemia, arthritis, hypertension and a variety of other diseases, has appeared in reputable medical journals in the U.S., France, Germany, Czechoslovakia, Russia, etc., since 1950. Extensive medical bibliographies have been compiled from time to time by the U.S. Library of Medicine (1960-1975).

"The dosage of EDTA for use in the treatment of sclerotic disease conditions, rate of administration, safety factors, toxicity and mechanism of action are well established in the American medical literature. Moreover, it has been estimated that more than 3,000 physicians in the U.S. have been involved in the clinical use of EDTA, primarily in the treatment of atherosclerosis or related disorders. It is further estimated that more than 200,000 patients have been treated in the U.S., involving more than one million individual treatments. Single persons have received over 500 treatments of EDTA over a period of ten years without ill effect. (Gordon and Vance, 1976.) EDTA has one of the best safety records of any medication used in the United States, with an LD_{50} of 2,000 mg/kg., making it 3.5 times less toxic than aspirin.

"Clinical symposia and workships are held twice a year under the aegis of the American Academy of Medical Preventics.* Standards of medical practice involving the use of EDTA are under continual review and updating by the AAMP. A review of the medical literature reveals that the practice of EDTA chelation therapy has been well established in the U.S. since the 1950s. The drug has received U.S.

---

*   The American Academy of Medical Preventics recently changed its name to the American College of Advancement in Medicine.

FDA acceptance in the past, and the efficiency, mechanism of action and safety factors are not new to the American medical community.

"This present bibliography of technical literature is substantial, and is more than merely 'anecdotal' in nature. A more comprehensive worldwide literature survey is now in progress by the AAMP and will be published at a later date."

The statement is signed as follows: Bruce W. Halstead, M.D., Member, Scientific Advisory Board, American Academy of Medical Preventics, 9 June 1976.

Dr. Halstead was subsequently elected to the presidency of AAMP, and brilliantly guided that organization to new heights. I was privileged to serve on the board of directors while he was president.

There are thirty-one pages of references in his book, *Chelation Therapy.*

It has become increasingly clear that as the human body ages, every cell accumulates more calcium than it should normally contain. This gums up the protoplasmic sap inside the cell, and prevents exchange of nutrients, wastes and beneficial products through the cell membrane.

Since the cell is the basic structural unit of every organ system, harmful consequences result to the entire organ system. If the kidney cells gum up, kidney disease results.

The circulatory system is the chief culprit in that it usually is the first to fail its mission—the adequate delivery of blood. The process is insidious and constant. Chronic disease results.

CHRONIC DEGENERATIVE ILLNESS

The frequency of chronic disorders has been increasing during the last three decades. This has been particularly evident in aging groups. The National Center for Health Statistics of the United States Public Health Service has noted that in the four year period from July 1957 to June 1961, an annual average of seventy-two million persons were reported to have one or more chronic disorders, diseases or impairments. Almost 20% of this population under fifteen years of age had one or more chronic disorders, whereas 80% of those over sixty-five were affected. Not only are death rates from chronic disease on the increase, but an additional thirty-eight million Americans suffer specifically from arthritis, rheumatism, mental illness and other impairments which do not enter into mortality statistics.

In 1960, physicians attending the Association of American Medical Colleges Teaching Institute in Hollywood Beach, Florida, were presented with a startling estimate of the prevalence of specific chronic diseases. Public Health Service statistics for the period July 1961 to June 1963 indicated that 80.3 million persons, or 44.1% of the civilian, noninstitutionalized population reported one or more chronic problems. For July 1963 to June 1964, the incidence had increased to 45.2% and for the period July 1964 to June 1965 an estimated 87.3 million persons or 46.3% of the civilian, noninstitutionalized population reported one or more chronic conditions or impairments. Thus within a span of four years there has been a 2.2% rise in the frequency of reported chronic disease.

Although not usually reported in the epidemiology of chronic disease, most health authorities readily concur that oral pathosis (abnormal tissue) is a major chronic problem in the United States. Doctor Wesley O. Young, in his contribution to the Commission on the Survey of Dentistry in the United States, summarized its enormity:

"The most obvious measure of the dental health problem is its sheer magnitude. It is estimated for example, that the 180 million people in the United States in the year 1960 have accumulated at least 700 million unfilled cavities. Diseases of the supporting bone and gingival tissues affect at least half of the population by the age of fifty and almost everyone by age sixty-five."

The eventual outcome of dental caries and peridontal disease is tooth loss. Statistics from the National Health Survey from 1960 through 1962 reveal that by sixty years of age, 35% of the American public is edentulous. They have lost all their natural teeth.

An important economic aspect of illness is the loss of manpower. According to figures cited by the United States Department of Health, Education and Welfare, the number of employed civilians absent from work on an average day in 1962 was 1.3 million. This amounted to 1.94% of the working civilian population. These values become even more significant when one realizes that not only is absenteeism greater today than in the 1950s, but that it prevails in spite of the continuing exponential rise in public and private expenditures for health and medical care. For example, total dollar outlay has swelled threefold in the past fifteen years.

Treating patients with multiple problems can be difficult when the physician has been practicing medicine with the "single shot" or "one thing at a time" philosophy. It's like handling quicksilver. No matter how hard one tries to confine it, there are always avenues of escape for the quicksilver.

If the treatment is done properly, all problem areas will be identified. Treatment will be tailored to support and rebuild these organ systems during the time the arteries and veins are being cleansed and reopened.

Because physicans on the whole do not practice this treatment does not infer that the treatment is too hard for the average doctor to learn. It is true that the treatment is not specific. It is not a short term procedure. Fluid medication entering the vein drop by drop circulates throughout the vascular system. This insures that all blood vessels, organs, organ systems and their protective wrappings of subcutaneous tissue, muscle, fat and skin, all nicely hung on a skeletal system of living bone, receive the nutrients and oxygen. As the inside diameter is cleansed and opened wider, more blood flows. Nutrition is boosted. Toxic wastes are removed more efficiently in less time.

When an old schoolmate or colleague asks me what we treat with EDTA chelation, I usually say, "The skin and its contents." Some of them have difficulty accepting that statement, but it is true nevertheless. There is no doubt the vascular system brings nourishment to every cell in the body, no matter where it may be. Is this not a better way to correct and reverse disease?

Reverend Robert Schuller, Garden Grove, California, has a thought I subscribe to heartily: "The most dangerous thing in the world is a negative-thinking expert."

14

The Importance of Diet and Vitamin Supplementation With Chelation Therapy

In their book, *Diet and Disease,* Doctor E. Cheraskin and his co-workers have extensively documented the relationship between nutrient intake from the food we eat and the prevention of chronic diseases. The inadequate dietary intake of essential nutrients is responsible for a great variety of serious chronic problems, and affects 50 to 75% of the population.

Not only are there millions of obviously ill people, but the morbidity figures from examinations of apparently healthy individuals present shocking evidence of what may be called silent sickness. A number of multiphasic examinations conducted on presumably healthy persons (Bolt 1955, Krehl 1964) have shown that those with newly discovered diseases range from 8.3 to 59.9%. This excludes previously known illness. When these two groups are combined, those designated as healthy are in the minority, namely 7.7 to 36.3%. Naturally, the more refined the testing procedures, the greater the disease yield. For example, replacing urinalysis by blood sugar studies (Thompson 1956) enhances the detection of abnormal carbohydrate metabolism by 61%.

When was the last time your doctor or his nurse took a detailed look at your food intake and its nutritional value?

Fully 50% of our food is processed and packaged before reaching the consumer. During the past two decades, the use of snack foods increased 80%; soft drinks, 80%; cakes and pastries, 60% and fast foods 100%. Nutritional deficiencies and errors are inevitable with such a dietary intake (*Wall Street Journal*, July 27, 1982.)

The failure to include nutritional appraisal in multiple testing programs has evoked much concern. Doctor Willare A. Krehl, Research Professor of Medicine and Director of the Clinical Research Center, State University of Iowa School of Medicine, discussed some of the reasons for this apathy toward nutrition in a recent article (1964):

"The nutritional evaluation of the patient is as important as any other aspect of the total evaluation. All too often one finds the patient is well-nourished and well-developed, or that the same patient seems to be getting a satisfactory diet. Alertness to the importance of nutritional well-being may have been dulled somewhat by the fact that frank deficiency disease such as scurvy, pellagra, beri-beri and rickets have largely disappeared. It is reasonable to assume, however, that nutritional deficiencies of all grades exist and do not necessarily appear as the florid evidence of the classical deficiency diseases. Just as atherogenesis and atherosclerosis commonly have a long silent course before coronary heart disease is clinically evident, so too one may have evidence of nutritional disease. The deficits may begin early in life and continue for long periods of time. They may contribute ultimately to an illness without themselves becoming identified as the cause of, or even related to, the illness."

The innovation of multiple testing that we do on every patient with chronic disease complaints, has unearthed much previously unrecognized diseases among so-called *healthy* people. The best way not to find early disease, of course, is not to look thoroughly.

On the other hand, there appears to be a true rise in chronic disorders, and we believe this can be reduced by proper diet and supplementation of nutrients not available in sufficient quantities to the patient because of loss by cooking, storage and the depletion of soil micronutrients. There has been a glaring failure to utilize nutritional testing procedures, not only in the ill but in examination of presumably well individuals.

Doctor T.D. Spies, formerly Professor of Nutrition and Metabolism, Northwestern Medical School, Chicago and Director, Nutritional Clinic, Hillman Hospital, Birmingham, Alabama, suggests the possibility of a nutritional factor in all disease:

"Today germs are not our principal enemy. Our chief medical adversary is what I consider a disturbance of the inner balance of the constituents of our tissues, which are built from and maintained by necessary chemicals in the air we breathe, the water we drink and the food we eat. For a generation we have worked on the concept that our cells are never static and that in time they must be replaced in varying degrees by the nutrients obtained from food. More specifically, our working hypothesis has been that all disease is chemical, and when we know enough, chemically correctable."

In the July 12, 1982 issue of *People* magazine, an article entitled, *In The War Against Cancer, The Latest Weapons are Fruit and Vegetables,* summarized the 445 page, two year report, *Diet, Nutrition and Cancer.*

The report, a study costing just under one million dollars, was prepared by the National Academy of Sciences. One of the report's thirteen authors, T. Colin Campbell, a professor of nutritional biochemistry of Cornell University, has been involved in cancer and diet research for seventeen years. He states in this interview that when fat intake increases, cancers of the colon, breast and prostate increase. Of all the dietary components studied, the evidence for a causal relationship between fat intake and cancer rise was most persuasive. He continues:

"There are various hypotheses. We don't know enough about any one of them. For colon cancer we do know that higher fat intake produces a higher level of certain bile acids in the gut. It turns out a couple of these bile acids are pretty good tumor promoters. If you give them to lab animals that you've given some carcinogens to, their chance of getting cancer is quite a bit greater."

Mr. Campbell details other healthful hints for a disease prevention food intake program. As the intake of beta-carotene increases the incidence of several types of cancer declines. This includes lung cancer. Beta-carotene is one of the yellow colored compounds called carotenoids. It is found in sweet potatoes, yellow vegetables, carrots, dark green vegetables and members of the cabbage family which include broccoli, kale, brussel sprouts and cauliflower. Beta-carotene is converted to vitamin A, which inhibits the cancer formation.

Whole grains are also recommended because they are a good source of fat-free energy, and contain beneficial amounts of fiber.

Richard S. Schweiker, Secretary of Health and Human Services, Washington, D.C., speaking at Rockefeller University said enough new data have emerged in recent, basic, clinical and epidemiologic studies to justify support for the hypothesis that micronutrients may prevent the initiation or development of cancer.

"This new strategy holds promise for reducing the incidence of cancer more successfully than an attempt to remove from the environment all substances which may initiate the cancer process—an approach which is not always possible or practical."

Characterizing the NCI program as a major example of "applied prevention," he said the new multimillion dollar studies are "focusing more on how we can interfere in the later stages of carcinogenesis to prevent cancer, instead of concentrating exclusively on substances which initiate the cancer process."

Secretary Schweiker also cited laboratory studies of vitamin A precursors (beta-carotene), vitamins C and E, selenium and certain chemicals demonstrating that these "act as preventive agents."

The National Cancer Institute program is also currently studying the role of vitamin C and vitamin E in other areas of cancer prevention. Dietary bran is getting a closer look as to its role in the prevention or recurrence of colorectal polyps, *Alpha tocopherol* (vitamin E) is being studied for its preventive role in fibrocystic disease of the breast.

At the request of the National Cancer Institute, a National Academy of Science task force looked at 10,000 studies in the medical literature. They concluded that the evidence is "increasingly impressive that cancers of most major sites are influenced by dietary patterns." The panel found that vitamins A, C and E appear to inhibit the promotion of cancer.

These recent findings should nail down the fact that vitamins are essential for good health, in spite of what some of the vociferous but misguided naysayers would have you believe.

An editorial from that same issue of *Medical Tribune* states in part:

"At long last our government has recognized the need to apply or put to objective and extensive tests the thesis of Linus Pauling and Roger J. Williams and yes, *Medical Tribune,* that the simple measure of improved nutrition, and the proper fortification with micronutrients, may enhance the health and extend the lifespan of Americans generally and be specific aids in the prevention and management of major common, disabling and deadly disorders. At long last a top government official speaks out to note that:

"In the laboratory, many of the micronutrients found in our diet—vitamin A precursors, vitamins C and E, selenium and certain chemicals—appear to act as cancer preventive agents. Laboratory studies are further strengthened by population studies which suggest that people who eat foods high in vitamin A or its precursor, beta-carotene, have fewer cancers of certain kinds, such as lung cancer, even if they have smoked cigarettes for a number of years."

In light of this official governmental recognition of the importance of disease prevention, and the fact that vitamins and minerals are indispensible for health, would it not be wise to advise the population to take oral supplements? A few tablets taken daily by the citizen is considerably less expensive than treatment of established disease later. In the long run, it's cheap insurance, and for twenty years we have witnessed its effectiveness.

Physicians interested in the elimination of disabling diseases such as arthritis, heart disease, diabetes, vascular disease and so forth, have found *through long experience that there are several common threads that weave themselves through all chronic debilitating conditions. Blood supply and proper nutrition are the most important of these, and they are inseparable, if one hopes to prevent, stop or reverse disability and dysfunction.* One of the problems is to determine just what each patient requires to balance his metabolic chemistry. A tailored program, made to fit each patient's unique requirements, is necessary. No two patients have the same chemical balance or deficiencies. Periodic re-examination is advised to *fine tune* and adjust dosages of nutrients.

A 1955 paper concluded:

– Large, often complete, deficiency of ascorbic acid frequently exists in arteries of apparently well nourished hospital autopsy subjects. Old age seems to accelerate the deficiency.

– Sections of atherosclerotic arteries had less ascorbic acid than adjacent non-atherosclerotic areas in the same artery.

– Scurvey in guinea pigs results in rapid onset of atherosclerosis. It has been reported that the aorta can manufacture cholesterol. The incorporation of radioactive acetate into cholesterol in tissue is said to be several times more rapid in tissues depleted of ascorbic acid.

– It is possible to correct the depletion in arteries by ascorbic acid therapy.

Another property of ascorbic acid is diuresis at high dosage levels (Evans 1938, Shaffer 1944). It will enable the body to remove excessive water retained in the tissues. This benefit is especially welcome when treating congestive heart failure, kidney diseases, or liver diseases that are characterized by swelling and water retention.

One of the early pioneers in the clinical use of megadoses of ascorbic acid is Dr. F.R. Klenner, Reedsville, North Carolina. He has used injected ascorbic acid for viral infections such as shingles, viral pneumonia, measles, chicken pox, mumps, influenza and polio myelitis (Klenner 1948, 1949). His results have been excellent.

Vitamin B-6 (pyridoxine) is added in amounts varying from 100 milligrams to 600 milligrams. This also aids in the elimination of excess water. Other beneficial effects at these elevated doses are the stabilization or irregular heart rhythms and improvement and elimination of joint pain in the arthritic patient. Using pyridoxine and ascorbic acid in effective dosage gets the job done with minimal electrolyte loss.

In his monograph, *The Justification for Vitamin Supplementation,* Dr. Jeffrey Bland talks of the effect that B-6 has on the structure and binding of glucocorticoid receptors. With two groups, Litwack et al. and Chidlowski (1979) demonstrated that B-6 will change or alter membrane binding efficiency of specific agents that respond to glucocorticoids. B-6 therefore may have an effect upon the function of adrenal gland hormones. This suggests that specific vitamin derived factors participate in membrane binding stability, and participate in the normalization of the endocrine system.

The adrenal gland hormones include Cortisol, etc. The effect of ACTH enhancement by vitamin B-6, therefore, is to enhance the body's ability to control and remove inflammation (enhancement of cortisol products). Arthritis inflammation and the inflammation associated with trauma, infections or allergic conditions are favorably managed.

Heparin may be added in cases where the patient is found to have excessive blood fats, and abnormal plethysmography (blood vessel tests showing loss of circulation due to narrowing of the inside diameter). Heparin thins the viscosity of the blood and helps dissolve fats that block the most important part of the vascular system, the microvasculature. These, the tiniest of vessels, nourish the most vital tissues.

In the cold of winter, you change to a thinner oil to insure good engine lubrication for your car. The motor starts and runs easier.

Once the viscosity of blood has been lowered in these vessels, nutrients and oxygen can penetrate deprived tissue. Dormant tissue cells are awakened and function improves.

Patients who have had heart attacks, senility, occlusive disease of the arteries leading to the brain, or gangrene might be given 5,000 units of heparin or more, per treatment. The dosage is adjusted according to laboratory test results. Blood test monitoring is done periodically.

Trace minerals analysis and supplementation is necessary for re-establishment of enzymes depleted or blocked by the chronic disease in progress. Without this step, the patient will not make speedy progress. Results will not be long-lasting. The patient will be tired, listless and fatigued. EDTA chelation therapy takes several minerals from the body—lead, calcium, copper, zinc, iron, cadmium and several others—depending upon the acidity or alkalinity of the solution and environment in which it is to function. Appropriate supplementation is necessary to achieve normal balance. Dr. Charles Rudolph has (with the aid of a programmer) set up our clinic's computer to do this for our patients. When the mineral analysis report is returned to us from the laboratory, the found values for the patient are fed into the computer, and a print-out lists the minerals that need to be supplemented. The dosage and time of day the pill is to be taken are stated also. It makes the doctor's job easier.

It is not the mission of this book to print multiple pages of menus for the reader. This information is available from physicians who are preventive minded. For the names of medical professionals in any area, inquiries should be addressed to the International Academy of Preventive Medicine or the American College of Advancement in Medicine. Either organization will be happy to provide the information patients need to interrupt that vicious cycle of deterioration and disability.

15

The Importance of Exercise With Chelation Therapy

No one has a right to live in idleness and expect to live long and be happy. The ship anchored in the harbor rots faster than the ship crossing the ocean; a still pool of water stagnates more rapidly than a running stream. Our unused muscles are subject to atrophy much more rapidly than those in use. The unused cells in our brains deteriorate much faster than those which are continually exercised. Hence, to remain young we must remain active.—Garth Henrichs

Heart function can be assessed and studied by means of treadmill testing. The patient taking a treadmill test walks on a horizontally leveled rubber belt that is driven at a set speed by an electric motor. The speed is quite slow at first, usually one mile per hour. Receptor wires for the electrocardiogram machine are attached to the chest of the patient. They remain in place throughout the test. Every three minutes an electrocardiograph tracing is run, making a permanent (hard data) record for later study by the doctor.

There is, in addition, a continuous display of the heart's activity on a television screen. This information is not permanent (soft data) because it is constantly changing as the test progresses. It provides, however, an instantaneous picture of heart activity as it is happening.

The speed of the moving belt and the angle of inclination are increased every three minutes. By increasing in standard increments, the angle or *grade of the hill* on which the patient must walk, the work-load on the heart is precisely determined. Changes in heart rate and blood pressure are measured, and the functional ability of the heart to do work is calculated.

The complete test consists of seven stages. The patient will have walked twenty-one minutes, and become more *uphill* at the same time.

A multistage stress electrocardiograph procedure is quite safe even for those with poor heart function. It is performed in small steps, each with its own cardiograph test. The physician will know by comparing these tracings from test to test, stage to stage, if problems are developing. The test will be stopped and corrective action taken if needed.

Data obtained from this procedure will give the physician a good appraisal of the patient's cardiac function, expressed as a percentage of normal function. We commonly see patients, for example, with varying percentages of impairment. A person could have an impairment of 42%, or 55% or 68%. Subtract this from 100%, and the actual functional ability of that person's heart to do work is determined.

A patient with an impairment of 42%, therefore, has 58% of the normally expected work capacity—42% subtracted from 100% is 58%. The fellow with 68% impairment is in serious trouble, for his functional ability is only 32%. We see patients in this state of serious cardiac impairment at the clinic quite frequently. Fortunately, they make outstanding recoveries.

It is not unusual for repeat treadmill tests taken at the conclusion of treatment to show 150% improvement. I never fail to be amazed and impressed with the ability of the most severely ill patients to make a return to health.

Several other types of information are provided by this method of testing. A multistage stress test done before and after treatment will show the improvement (or lack of improvement) caused by that treatment.

It would be interesting to compare the treatments used to-day by other physicians to EDTA chelation therapy. Any clinical or scientific test can be used, but perhaps the maximum multistage stress electrocardiogram test, just described, would be a good place to start. Patients treated with EDTA would be shown to benefit many times more, when compared to those treated with drugs or surgery.

McDonagh Medical Center has shown repeatedly that this form of treatment reduces and prevents the atherosclerotic buildup of fats and cholesterol (1981, 1982). The treatment can open the narrowed inside diameters of plugged arteries as proved by another paper published by our group entitled: *An Occulocerebrovasculometric Analysis of the Effect of EDTA Chelation Upon Vascular Stenosis.*

Mr. Doug Wussow, the director of Midwest Health and Livestyle, Kansas City, Missouri has been closely observing our patients for the past several years. His training in exercise physiology and cardiac rehabilitation qualifies him to prescribe the type and frequency of exercise most beneficial to our patients. Close perusal by Mr. Wussow has led to the collection and presentation of sufficient data to assemble eight papers for the medical literature. Some salient findings are presented here.

Seventy-three patients were included in one investigation. The subjects were divided into two groups, exercisers taking EDTA chelation treatment (thirty-four in number), and non-exercisers taking EDTA chelation treatment (thirty-nine in number). All subjects underwent two maximal multistage stress tests on a motor driven treadmill, one prior to beginning the treatment and one at the end of the treatment program. The results are as follows:

Heart rate. It was found that the maximal heart rate went up slightly in the exercise and EDTA chelation group (5%), and remained unchanged in the non-exercise EDTA chelation group. At three submaximal workloads, the heart rate went down in both groups 5 to 9%, but the decrease was greater in the exercise and EDTA chelation group.

METS (work capacity). It was found that the maximal work capacity went up significantly in both groups. In the exercise group taking EDTA therapy, it was 37.5%. In those taking EDTA therapy, but not exercising, it was 16.0%.

Rate pressure product, (RPP). The maximal RPP was found to be unchanged in both groups. The submaximal RPP went down 10 to 18%, but it was consistently greater in the exercising EDTA group.

Systolic blood pressure (SBP). Submaximal SBP went down 10.6% in the exercise and EDTA group, and 6.1% in the non-exercise and EDTA group. The maximal SBP remained unchanged in both groups.

Dyastolic blood pressure (DBP). Maximal DBP went down 9.8% in the exercise and chelation group. Submaximally DBP was reduced 5 to 11% in both groups with the exercise and EDTA chelation group's decrease being consistently greater than the other group.

S-T depression. S-T segment depression was reduced 46% in both groups during maximal exercise. The rate of positive tests (S-T depression greater than 1 mm) was reduced 50% in both groups.

These findings are consistent with the great clinical improvement seen in EDTA chelation patients who do aerobic exercises. The heart shows significant improvement in its ability to function normally again. Results are outstanding, and cannot be attained by the usual treatment offered heart patients in this country today. This high quality of improvement cannot be achieved without EDTA chelation treatment and the inclusion of aerobic conditioning through a prescribed, monitored program.

Some type of aerobic (non-stop) exercise is a must. The condition of many patients will not permit much exercise at first, but eventually they will have made enough progress to begin. This type of exercise greatly multiplies the chelation effect.

Twenty years ago, before utilization regulation was devised, I put all chelation patients in the hospital. We did thirty treatments in thirty days. The patient was then given a month to rest, and then the thirty day treatment cycle was repeated. I did frequent testing then, because I was learning the treatment. One of the reasons doctors have difficulty learning EDTA chelation therapy is the inability to follow a patient's progress by hospitalization and frequent testing.

After eighteen months or so, the utilization restriction procedures were put into effect by the government for Medicare patients. A patient could no longer stay in the hospital for extended treatment. The government would not pay. New chelation patients were then treated in the office. After another year, I compared results.

I was amazed to learn that the hospitalization patients, with their controlled diet, medicine schedule, etc., took longer to get results than office treated patients.

It took 33% more treatments for hospitalized patients. When I began to search the records for the reason, it became apparent that the only difference was the exercise factor. Hospitalized patients didn't get the small, but regular, amount of movement that my office patients did. Just the usual daily routine of the ambulatory patient made this gigantic difference.

At that time exercise was prescribed. Aerobic exercise is the most efficient. Patients are monitored electronically, and heart rate and rhythm is closely observed. The patient's progress is enhanced even more than we originally expected.

16

At the Clinic

Patients who come in from out of state, and there are many, must find their own living accomodations. There are several motels nearby, and of course, Kansas City has many good hotels.

The flat-roofed, 16,000 square foot building that houses McDonagh Medical Center was built three years ago. It sets on a gently sloping lot so that parking is available on two levels. There are entrances on both levels.

A new patient will find the first day busy indeed. He will be asked to fill out the usual health history questionnaire, and several tests are given to help evaluate the patient's mental and psychological state. Unless there is a special preference, the patient will be assigned to a physician, who will be in charge of his case.

If he has been fasting overnight, the patient will be taken to the laboratory where blood will be drawn for blood chemistry testing. Testing will be done for serum calcium, phosphorus, iron, magnesium, sodium, potassium, chlorides, BUN, creatinine, glucose, uric acid, cholesterol, triglycerides, thyroid function, several enzymes, liver function and glycohemoglobin. Prostatic acid phosphate is done on all male patients to detect early prostate changes.

In addition to checking organ function through blood chemistries, a complete blood count with white blood cell differential is done. To screen the patient for precancerous changes in the gastrointestinal system, a blood test called CEA is performed.

If indicated by the patient's history, food allergy tests are made. These may include skin tests, sublingual testing, or cytotoxic testing.

Cytotoxic testing is an interesting procedure. White blood cells are separated from the whole blood, and diluted. A drop of white blood cell solution is mixed on a glass slide with a drop of the appropriate food solution. Foods are selected on the basis of a frequency questionnaire. If the patient admits to a frequency of ingestion of the suspected food (likely to cause allergy reaction), a test with that food is performed. The white cells will disintegrate when the test is positive. I have watched them under the microscope, and they virtually explode before your eyes.

Depending on the number of cells that break up in a certain measured period of time, the allergy can be graded as to its severity. For example, the destruction of four or more cells may be graded 3 +, two cells destroyed may be called 2 +, and so on.

A criticism of this test procedure is made by those who either do not do the test properly, and hence get unreliable results, or by people who have an economic interest in doing allergy testing the long, hard, expensive way.

Properly performed by a knowledgeable technician using fresh living white cells, the test has proved its worth. It is not a blood test that can be sent off to an outside lab. After a few hours the cells will not be viable when finally tested, and results will be worthless.

TREATMENT PROCEDURE

Once the decision is made to begin chelation therapy, a treatment schedule is set up to obtain the best results in the shortest possible time. This will vary, depending on the patient, the pathological problems exhibited, the patient's age and personal preferences. It takes on the average of thirty to forty bottles of fluid dripped slowly at first, probably for three to four hours or more. After we determine the individual tolerance to the flow rate, and after the patient has had several bottles, the flow rate often can be reduced.

If the patient takes a treatment on an empty stomach, about one in twenty people will experience some nausea. In order to prevent this we ask each patient to eat immediately before starting each treatment. Some of them will also bring food such as crackers, fresh fruit, hard boiled egg whites, etc., to eat during the infusion period.

EDTA is put into a liter (nearly a quart) of fructose solution. A small amount of procaine is sometimes added to keep the vein from becoming irritable and painful. Most people do not require procaine, however. B complex vitamins and heparin to remove fats from the vessel wall are sometimes added if blood tests indicate too many blood fats. To monitor progress, certain blood tests may be repeated depending on the initial blood picture. The patient does not have to lay down for treatment. Some sit in a chair and read, write letters, or perform light work. However, some patients do prefer to lie down and take a nap. Almost all of our patients sit in an easy chair and watch television. Some patients want privacy, so we put them in a room by themselves. All patients are closely monitored throughout the infusion time.

HYPERBARIC OXYGEN

Hyperbaric oxygen therapy (HBO) is available to the most seriously ill patients, or those who might want to accelerate their recovery. This extra boost to the healing process is remarkable. I would compare the difference to that of a jet fighter aircraft when the pilot turns on his afterburner. It really multiples the speed.

In some cases, HBO is prescribed. In some cases not as critical, it is optional. In the booklet entitled *Hyperbaric Oxygen Therapy,* a detailed explanation of this therapy is presented. The booklet is written for the patient, and is easily understood. It gives the patient a basic understanding of the use of HBO treatment of such chronic degenerative diseases as atherosclerosis, coronary heart disease, senility, peripheral vascular (circulation) diseases and other disorders.

Wasting diseases such as multiple sclerosis are responding to the combination of EDTA chelation, nutrient supplementation, food allergy and dietary control and hyperbaric oxygen. While true cures may not be claimed, I feel there is a remarkable breakthrough just over the horizon.

A paper showing the effect of HBO on multiple sclerosis was presented by Dr. B. Fischer, M.D. at the Conference on Clinical Application of Hyperbaric Oxygen. He did a double blind study on a series of MS patients using only HBO. Half of the patients received 100% oxygen pressurized to twice that of the atmosphere. The control patients received a mixture of air that was pressurized the same way, but contained the amount of oxygen normally available in the atmosphere.

Both groups were given twenty treatments, at which point therapy was ended. All patients were observed for one year with frequent examinations. The conclusions of the study were startling. Those treated with HBO achieved remission or great improvement, and maintained it very nicely. All patients were able to function better, and some were able to return to work. Control subjects made no improvement, and during a twelve month follow-up period deteriorated. They had more functional loss than was present before the study began. The data are highly significant, and published in the January 1983 issue of the *New England Journal of Medicine.*

GETTING THOSE RESULTS

In order to make the treatment as efficient as possible, several accessory procedures are available to patients. Some are routine and some are ordered at the discretion of the treating physician. Naturally the severity of the patient's condition is important, and the more compromised the patient's condition, the more big guns we bring to bear. The mixture of ingredients and fluids for intravenous administration are variable. They are tailored as much as possible to fit a patient's laboratory and testing characteristics.

No two patients will have the same blood chemistries or the same amount of vascular occlusion. Many people have multiple illnesses. A survey of our patient records have revealed that the average patient seen at McDonagh Medical Center has eight diagnoses. Dr. E. Cheraskin, M.D., who heads our research department, made the survey.

A typical patient's history is as follows:

Patient: M.L.R., age 51, male.

Present illness or complaint: Headaches, tiredness, loss of pep and energy, sex problems, circulation, lungs and breathing, stomach and swallowing, muscles or joints, eyes, nose, throat, or mouth, nervousness, pain, needs a check-up. (This information was written by the patient when completing his diagnostic health profile questionnaire.)

Social history: Married. No children. U.S. citizen, born in the United States.

Religion: Protestant.

Occupation: Employed, a trade.

Military: Yes.

Family Medical History: Definite diabetes in grandparents. Heart disease in mother. Gout in brother or sister. Arthritis in other blood relatives.

General Information: Believe symptoms have occurred as the result of industrial exposure. Has been exposed to dust, fumes, chemicals, paints, lacquers, varnishes, excessive heat, excessive cold. Some exposures occur at work.

Immunizations and Vaccinations: Polio (three sugar cubes), smallpox, typhoid, tetanus booster received within last ten years. Illness: mumps.

Nutritional: Now on restricted diet for other unlisted condition. Eats three meals. Eats between meals, at bedtime. Daily diet—meat, vegetables, dairy products, salads, grains.

Eyes: Has poor vision. Progressively worse in spite of glasses.

Ears: No positive responses.

Mouth, Nose, Throat: No positive responses.

Past and Present Drug Reactions: Has had drug reaction to other unlisted medications. Thinks some symptoms may be due to drug reactions.

Energy and Weight: Weight at age 20 was 155 pounds. Weight at age 40 was 199 pounds. Present weight 179 pounds. In past year has lost by dieting. Excessive fatigue. Lacks energy and strength. Wakes up tired. Tires easily. Is tired by afternoon. Feels constantly tired. Tiredness is moderate. Tiredness is physical, emotional, both physical and emotional.

Hematology (blood and malignancy): No positive response.

Thyroid: Cold intolerance. Feels cold when others are not. Has to wear more clothing than others.

Other Indocrine: Generalized hair loss. Skin has become lighter. Has been given steroids. Twenty-four hour fluid intake less than three quarts. Has had unexplained sweating. Has stretch marks.

Diabetes and Hypoglycemia: When hungry has weakness, dizziness, light headedness, restlessness, difficulty thinking. Has had glycosuria (sugar in urine) on routine examination. Has had hypoglycemia. (Abnormal elevation in blood sugar.) Previous glucose tolerance test borderline. Previous diagnosis of borderline diabetes.

Diabetes Treatment: Has been treated for abnormal glucose tolerance. Has taken oral antidiabetic medication.

Skin (Dermatology): Has had recurrent other unlisted skin infections. Located on face. Has cutaneous mass, which is enlarging, tender. Has had unexplained itching. Has had many brown pigment spots on skin.

Allergy: Has experienced hives. Allergy symptoms seem caused by dust, certain smells, flowers, grasses. Has had sinusitis, sinus drainage, sinus congestion, sniffling, post-nasal drip, nasal congestion, nasal drainage, nasal polyps, frequent sneezing, spells of sneezing, mouth breathing, loss of smell, loss of taste. Symptoms occur mostly at random. Has sore throat in the morning. Has popping and/or congestion in ears. Smokers in family. Symptoms aggravated by winter heating, cold fronts, rain and dampness, dryness. Gets allergy symptoms from grapefruit. Has used Chlortrimaton, Ornade. Uses a few decongestants frequently. Uses nose drops or spray daily. Air conditioning is central refrigerated unit. Heating is central hot air. Fails to change filters regularly. Carpet pads are foam rubber. Bedroom curtains are synthetic. Bedspread is synthetic fiber. Pillows are feather, dacron.

Respiratory (Lungs): Has had positive tuberculin test. Previous chest x-ray was abnormal. Dyspneic (short of breath) at rest, with usual exertion. Avoids exertion because of dyspnea. After twenty stair steps is dyspneic. Smokes cigarettes. Has intermittent cough. Cough is moderate. Expectorates very little. Wheezes at rest, with colds, on exertion, with deep breathing, on talking, after coughing. Wheezes on exposure to dust, fumes, smoke, certain chemicals.

Cardiovascular: Dizzy when arising from sitting. Dizzy when arising from lying. Occurs rarely. On walking legs get exceedingly tired. Has coldness of hands, feet.

Gastrointestinal: Has had surgery on appendix. Usually has bowel movement daily. Never uses a laxative. Has had blood in stool. Has had hemorrhoids, treated by surgery.

Urinary section: Has nocturia (night urination), frequently. Potency problem is associated with depression, marital discord, reduced libido, inability to ejaculate. Has had vasectomy. Sterility has been verified.

Arthritis: Has had unexplained recurrent leg pain, generalized discomfort, hurts all over, chest tenderness, symptoms have increased. **Check costosternal joints.** Symptoms have increased. Symptoms are worse with damp weather, with cold weather, with temperature change. Symptoms are worse at night. Now taking medication for arthritis. Has arthritic symptoms in shoulders, elbows, wrists, hands, fingers, chest, sternum, neck, back, dorsal spine, coccyx, hips, knees, ankles, feet, toes. Has had rheumatoid arthritis, traumatic arthritis, septic arthritis. Has taken arthritis medication with improvement. Joint tenderness is moderate, severe, persistent, intermittent, unpredictable. Has had arthralgia for no apparent reason. Early morning stiffness. Has had acute arthritis of hands (possible chiragra), feet (possible podagra), larger joints.

Neuromuscular: Has unexplained difficulty walking, limping, loss of balance, sleepiness, light headedness, clumsiness, muscular weakness.

Psychological: Has spells of depression. Afraid of failure. Sleeps poorly. Uses alcohol rarely. Wants to discuss emotional problems. Is more irritable.

Headaches: Symptoms occur weekly, occasionally. Location usually generalized. Now taking medication for headaches. Headaches are longstanding. Intensity is usually moderate, severe. Previous diagnosis of histamine headache. Symptoms associated with emotional tension, fatigue, frustration, travel. Headache usually associated with neck ache.

Marital: Disagrees with spouse concerning money. Has been married more than twenty-five years. Marriage problems cause tension, nervousness, overeating...Other problems or tensions cause overeating. Happily married. Married once. Spouse has been married once.

Medications: Now taking medication for arthritis, headaches.

Surgeries: Has had surgery of appendix, anal surgery, vasectomy.

History Symptoms: Has had reaction to other unlisted medications. Thinks some symptoms are due to drug reactions. Lacks energy. Lacks strength. Has had glycosuria on routine examination. Has had hypoglycemia. Previous diagnosis of borderline diabetes. Has had an enlarging cutaneous mass. Has tender, cutaneous mass. Has had positive tuberculin test. Previous abnormal chest x-rays. Dyspneic at rest. Dyspneic with usual exertion. Avoids exertion because of dyspnea. Dizzy on arising from lying. Has had blood on stool. Has had acute arthritis of hands (possible chiragra). Has had acute arthritis of feet (possible podagra). Has unexplained difficulty walking. Has unexplained limping. Has unexplained sleepiness. Has unexplained loss of balance. Has unexplained light-headedness. Has unexplained clumsiness. Has unexplained muscular weakness. Wants to discuss emotional problems.

This is just an "average" patient history that we commonly see at the clinic. Many of them are in considerably worse health. Many have advanced occlusive disease of the blood vessels, and at the same time may be suffering from disease of the liver, eyes, kidneys, heart and lungs. Diabetes and senility are common also.

The patient history files at our clinic cover a section of wall twenty-five feet long, from floor to ceiling. Of the many thousands of file folders, probably 25% are case histories of people who have had gangrene, in addition to other diseases.

All of them have had excellent reversal of the disease pro-cess in the arteries, and the patients were saved from the horrors of amputation: loss of function, forced retirement or loss of unemployment, and the psychological terror of being an incomplete or crippled individual.

The patients and their families were suddenly forced, by the reality of amputation, to make adjustments in their life-style.

Perhaps the worst case that I can recall was a diabetic man, Mr. X, age seventy, who had advanced vascular disease in both legs. Both feet were dark maroon in color, swollen, infected and draining from the toenails. There were two or three black gangrenous toes on each foot. He had hy-pertension, visual loss, kidney disease and cerebral vascular insufficiency (senility). His was a difficult case indeed.

This man had five children, three boys and two girls. Both of the girls were nurses. Each week he was under treatment, one son and one daughter stayed with him to provide care and nursing. A family friend had advised them to have EDTA chelation treatment and perhaps save his legs from amputation. The patient was in the hospital at the time and the surgeons were going to operate in two days' time. The patient and his family decided that the surgery could always be done if chelation did not work, and so he was checked out of the hospital, and flown across two states to be seen one morning at our clinic.

His appearance was bad. He was very thin, and his face had a washed out gray color to it, the expression showing the pain he suffered. He was tired and could barely maintain his posture in the wheelchair. He wanted to slouch and let his head fall forward several times during the brief interview.

We prescribed an extended treatment plan, characterized by several weeks of treatment, a few weeks' rest, then more treatment. As usual, we were able to gradually reduce his in-sulin dosage. He made a good recovery, and could once again walk and enjoy his retirement.

The earliest case of gangrene that I can remember treating with EDTA was also advanced, and difficult to treat. The pa-tient, Mr. G.S., was a man in his sixties who smoked three packages of cigarettes daily, and had an alcohol problem. He lived alone, and judging by his asthenic frame, ate irregularly and unwisely.

Entering the treatment room, I was overwhelmed by the terrible smell of rotting flesh that filled the room. The patient sat in a chair, resting his right foot on a small stool. Bandages over the ball of the foot, and toes, were wet with yellow-staining pus.

The man was in great pain, as judged by the way he moved. His face mirrored the great amount of pain he suffered. The man was not able to concentrate or give a coherent history of his illness. His temperature was 103.5 F. I sent him to a hospital located in a small town near Kansas City. It was 1962, and some of the smaller hospitals would allow EDTA chelation treatment at that time. Medicare had not yet put utilization rules into effect.

After the usual testing and x-rays had been done, EDTA chelation therapy was begun. The patient, a diabetic, had a resistant infection in the gangrenous foot, and also one in his kidneys. His temperature elevation persisted for five or six days. Two of his toes sloughed spontaneously. Slowly, the combination of hospital care, regular feedings, appropriate antibiotics and EDTA treatment began to take effect. Three weeks later, the patient was walking down the hall with the aid of crutches.

Following his discharge from the hospital, he continued treatment in the office, and made a complete recovery.

A short time later, following a monthly hospital staff meeting, I had an interesting conversation with the chief of staff of the hospital, and the chief of surgery. They wanted to discuss this case, and marveled at the recovery made by this patient. The surgeon called the chief of staff to observe the patient daily. Both of them watched his chart, and examined the patient. They were positive the case would go "sour" and they would order amputation.

Cases of early, or minor gangrene, as we have come to call it, are hardly worth telling about. They respond with no difficulty, and are easy to treat. There have been hundreds of these cases, too.

17

Just How Important Is Chelation Therapy?

Chelation therapy is very important for a number of reasons. To understand why chelation is so effective let's define the process once again.

Since the arteriosclerotic process is generally considered to be a constantly deteriorating disease, it is gratifying to see patients continue to improve over the years. A note of sadness is always present in the minds of chelating physicians when they realize that the vast multitude of patients needing chelation will not receive it because their physicians either don't know about it, or are prejudiced against it.

The surgical approach cannot provide anything beyond temporary relief. It is stop gap and superficial. After one or two surgical bypasses, the patient is abandoned, because nothing more can be done surgically. He simply dies, or lives with increased limitations. Frequently vascular surgery offers only symptomatic relief from pain.

Medicine in general has a poor batting average when it comes to effective treatment and reversal of chronic illness in any case. In fact, modern medicine strikes out more than it should.

EDTA treatment can make the difference. Life can be lived fully, and disease already present reversed. Those with little or no disease can be offered life-long avoidance of disease. Surgeries and/or chronic medical treatment can be avoided.

The reversal and prevention of the leading killer diseases, those chronic debilities that relentlessly worsen in spite of all the "stop gap" treatments—drugs or surgical procedures that modern medicine can offer—is not impossible. It is not particularly difficult either. For the vast majority of patients, treatment is done without drugs. This comes to only 10 to 15% of the cost of bypass surgery. It works, and it works well.

Readers who would like copies of the published papers we have produced attesting to the efficacy of EDTA chelation treatment may request them from McDonagh Medical Center, 2800 Kendallwood Parkway, Kansas City, Missouri, 64119.

There are many studies which have challenged the efficacy of coronary bypass surgeries. Here is one that is indicative of the average effectiveness of these costly procedures:

In 1984, the *New England Journal of Medicine* published a study of eighty-two patients who had endured one or more bypass operations and who had survived the operation one year. The one year survival norm is used to designate an operation a *success.*

The study originally included one-hundred forty-eight patients, and eighty-two of them were re-examined after ten years. The others were not examined because nine of them were older than seventy-five years, and eighteen had vascular problems too severe to permit the study. Others were not studied for personal reasons not relevant to our discussion. We are not told how many of the patients who lived one year—and were thus selected for study—died before the ten year period was up. Nor are we told how they died.

Ten years later 31% of the eighty-two patients were unchanged. The remaining patients had further progression of the vascular disease.

This means 48% of the eighty-two patients had noticeable further narrowing of their blood vessels, including the grafts; 21% of the eighty-two patients had *total obstruction* of at least one bypass graft.

To say it another way, 69% of the surviving eighty-two patients who lived ten years after a bypass operation had serious problems of continuing deterioration. Only 31% of these patients could be defined as having no additional problems following the bypass operations.

I have many other studies which show the success rate even lower. I have never found a treatment that provides as much improvement to the vascular patients as does EDTA chelation therapy. This is my considered opinion and experience. Yet today people who are ill are having their medical rights denied. As a consequence, they are dying needlessly early of strokes, heart attacks and other chronic problems.

An outstanding paper has been published by H. Richard Casdorph, M.D. Dr. Casdorph is currently Assistant Clinical Professor of Medicine at the University of California Medical School, Irving, California. He received his training in cardiovascular diseases at Mayo Clinic and earned his Ph.D. in medicine from the University of Minnesota. More recently he has taught at UCLA Medical School and has been Chief of Medicine at Long Beach Community Hospital.

Doctor Casdorph included eighteen patients in his report. All had documented arteriosclerotic heart disease. They were studied using the isotope Technetium 99m to measure left ventricular ejection fraction before and after the administration of EDTA chelation therapy. A statistically significant improvement in left ventricular ejection fraction occurred in this group of patients, proving that EDTA chelation therapy returns diseased heart function to normal.

Scientific studies published by our clinical group have shown that EDTA chelation therapy is an effective treatment. Many times it has been life-saving. We have shown the treatment lowers high blood cholesterol and blood fats, opens occluded arteries, lowers high blood pressure, smooths irregular heartbeats and improves kidney function.

Intravenous fluid itself is important in this treatment modality. If the patient is low in sodium, or in chloride, saline or half-normal saline should be used for the vehicle. Other patients require distilled water, dextrose solutions, or other intravenous solutions. When possible we use a liter (1,000 cc). Some chelating physicians use half that volume (500 cc) to transport the EDTA and other ingredients. We feel that a full liter will reduce blood viscosity, inflate and perfuse the capillary network of blood vessels more efficiently. More volume is perfused to absorb, dissolve and carry away toxins. If you were to flush out the radiator of your automobile, you would want to use plenty of water.

EDTA DOSAGE

To the solution vehicle one to three grams of ethylenediaminetetracetic acid are added. For patients with severe multiple problems, the initial dosage might be reduced to a fraction of one gram. When progess is seen in the blood chemistries, the dosage of EDTA is gradually raised until the maximal dosage of three grams per treatment is attained.

Doctors using chelation successfully in the battle against chronic disease are practicing their skill at the cutting edge of medicine. It is an exciting, satisfying way to truly salvage human lives. Helping a patient that has been told there is no hope for further progress gives a feeling of fulfillment as nothing else can. I would not trade places with anyone on this earth.

All of the doctors at our clinic have told me they feel the same way. Patients see it in the attitude of the physicians. They frequently remark, "You fellows have fun practicing medicine, don't you?" (As if it might be illegal!) The thirty or so employees have the same attitude, with a ton of concern, loyalty and elbow grease thrown in. In short, they care. They are happy for the tremendous improvements in patients, especially when they have a part in a patient's progress.

The product of any good medical system is health, or wellness. Is the American system short-changing the paying public of its health product because of a superficial, less-than-responsible health care policy?

Every solid, finished product must stand on its own. Ideally, it will function trouble-free, requiring a minimum of maintainence. To do this, it had to be investigated thoroughly, tested time and again to prove its worth, then finally assembled.

To have a first class product, all other considerations must be secondary. The winds of politics, cost manipulation and personal prejudices must not be allowed to bend the concept of the finished design. To do otherwise will insure our approach being other than first class.

I don't believe there is any argument that keeping our citizens in good health is good for our country. It has been said that a first class health care program is too costly. Not so! Properly done, a high degree of wellness lasts indefinitely. This would be much less costly than the present system. Conventional medicine treats the top of the iceberg only, and underlying diseases keep popping up repeatedly in the patient, only to necessitate more (and costly) treatment and use of in-patient facilities and skilled personnel. When greed and commercialization creep in to influence the method of keeping our populace healthy, there is a cost problem. Vested interests must take their profits. Their profits decline as the health of the nation increases. Is this happening in the United States?

It is better to treat and reverse disease at the earliest possible time. Our should we wait until it's bad enough, then bypass the coronary arterial occlusion, or amputate the leg?

Those with chronic disease should take more responsibility in the battle for health. They can reasonably expect to benefit from proper food intake, supplementation of nutrients and exercise. Continued cost escalation and bodily deterioration is their future if continued dependence on ineffective treatment and drug therapy is their sole treatment method.

Many of the most seriously ill patients who are seen in our clinic for the first time are usually taking several drugs. Some of them are in poor or fair control of their illness, even though they may be taking twenty or more pills and capsules daily. And what of the cost?

According to a recent article in *Wall Street Journal,* the nation's health care bill has increased more than 15% to $287 billion per annum. The Health Care Financing Administration said the federal government's share of health-care spending last year was $84 billion and state and local governments spent $39 billion. Combined outlays equaled

43% of the total spent on health care, the agency said.

A reduction of this enormous cost to our population is mandatory. With EDTA chelation therapy, nutrient supplementation, continuing aerobic exercises and proper food selection, patients can expect to reduce their health care costs. It is possible to reduce the great costs by half or more, and this estimate is conservative.

People must be educated in these methods. They must take command of their health and not delegate that care to health professionals who may or may not have the proper dedication, knowledge and motivation.

How can one not become enthusiastic about a treatment method that will return normal body function, stop deterioration and give improvement in physical and mental energy? This method will enable you to live a longer, healthier life and to top it all: it saves money.

Several years ago, I had the good fortune to be invited to a dinner by a very unusual gentleman. He had what many of us might think was a terrible handicap. His speech was impaired due to a birth defect. He had a cleft palate.

He didn't believe he had a liability. He believed this to be a golden opportunity. He thought people would listen to him with concentration and attention. He was correct.

During the five years that I followed Glen Turner's career, his cosmetic company grew with the speed of a moon rocket. His personal fortune was said to be in excess of $300 million.

One of the things he used to say repeatedly to people is a thought that is pertinent to this book. When people would ask how he was able to build a company (and his personal fortune) in such a short time and with no background in the business, he'd say, "Hard jobs are done by those who can, but impossible jobs are done by those who care." This is a powerful statement full of meat for all of us—young, old and in between.

Many patients come to our clinic after making the "grand tour" of some of the country's most famous hospitals. Usually they are given surgical procedures, placed on several drugs and told they cannot expect to make any more progress. They have believed there was no hope of regaining health and vigor. Normal function was to be denied them for the rest of their shortened lifespan. Fortunately, this is usually not true. They have been able to regain normal function and live life fully, in the mainstream again.

One such case comes to mind. A Mennonite farmer, age sixty-nine, came to inquire about the treatment he had heard about. He had been released from the hospital in his home state about ten days before. He was suffering from shortness of breath, increasing chest pain and great swelling in the feet and legs. He had been released after three weeks of hospitalization with diagnosis of hypertension (high blood pressure), coronary artery disease and congestive heart failure. Secondary diagnoses included kidney disease and peripheral vascular disease of arteriosclerotic origin (hardening of the arteries in his arms and legs).

The arteries in his heart, kidneys and legs were narrowed with calcium. At 298/140 his blood pressure was dangerously elevated. He could not lace his shoes. Swollen tissue protruded over both shoe tops.

This gentleman was treated for one week with intravenous EDTA daily. Therapy was then reduced to three treatments per week for another two months. His blood pressure normalized. He went back to his farm and could load hay bales with his farmhands following the completion of treatment. The four drugs he took three times daily that had originally been ordered by the hospital physician were reduced to two tablets daily.

Another case is typical of our experience every day at the clinic:

Mr. I.M., age sixty-three, an engineer by profession, suffered a heart attack while shoveling snow several years ago. He was placed in the CCU under the care of his family physician, who happened also to be chief of internal medicine and cardiology at a local hospital. The patient's condition finally stabilized after a prolonged, rocky course. His heart arrested twice, requiring emergency electroshock to restart.

He was finally discharged in stable condition, and was placed on five drugs to maintain his heart and blood pressure. His physician referred him to another hospital in Kansas City to have coronary arteriography. In this procedure, a thin catheter (tube) is inserted into an artery in the arm or leg and worked upstream to the heart's coronary arteries. Dye is then injected, and a series of X-rays are taken. If the artery being studied is occluded, a diminished amount of dye will pass the point of occlusion.

This test indicated that the left anterior descending coronary artery (the main artery of the heart) was occluded 90% or more, and there were two other major coronary arteries that had 50 to 70% blockage. The patient was told he would not live more than three months if he did not submit to coronary bypass surgery.

At this point he came to McDonagh Medical Center, and I interviewed him for the first time. He seemed to know quite a bit about EDTA chelation therapy, including the pharmacology, method of treatment, mechanism of action and the early history of the treatment in this country. As this first meeting progressed, his questions became more technical. When he asked about the minute biochemical details—how the molecular activity was sustained, or what determined the preference of the molecule for the various metals removed, it became apparent that he was as knowledgeable about EDTA as I. I said, "Mr. M, I'm more interested in the clinical application of this treatment, as we have the majority of our experience there. I might not have the answers you want, but my partner, Dr. Rudolph, can give them to you. He holds a Ph.D. in biochemistry, as well as a medical degree."

"I appreciate your frankness, Doctor," he said. "If you would have lied to me I'd have caught you. You see, this is information close to my field of work. I went to the medical library and reseached EDTA before I came here. Your clinic has treated several people from our company, and that is how I became aware of the good results your patients get. I will take this treatment."

This man was examined and found to have severe coronary occlusive disease and peripheral vascular disease. The arteries in the thighs, calves and ankles were occluding. The carotid arteries in the neck were also plugging up and he was in danger of a stroke. He could not walk more than thirty feet without pain in his chest, radiating down the left arm. Walking caused him to wince with pain and clutch the left side of his chest. His facial color was ash-gray and he could walk no further.

Uric acid, serum cholesterol, BUN and creatinine (kidney function), triglyceride and liver function were abnormally high. His blood pressure was elevated. A treadmill electrocardiogram procedure showed very poor heart function. The test had to be stopped after two minutes due to t-wave inversion greater than 1mm. This indicated his coronary arteries could not deliver the necessary blood to sustain this amount of physical work.

He required nitroglycerine tablets six to ten times daily to control the chest pain. Medication had been prescribed for sleep and to calm him during the day. He had been advised not to drive his car. His doctor feared the stress of rush hour traffic would be too much strain for his heart.

This gentleman was started on intravenous EDTA. Dietary changes to minimize fat, sugar, salt and alcohol intake were advised. Food allergies were determined and the patient advised as to how to avoid them. Trace mineral analysis indicated several mineral imbalances. The patient was placed on a corrective mineral supplementation program. Vitamin supplementation, orally and as an inclusion in the intravenous bottle was begun. Vitamin E, B complex, pyridoxine, thiamin, ascorbic acid, potassium, magnesium, zinc and other supplements were tailored to his needs.

After the fourth treatment, he remarked that his chest pain was greatly improved. By the third month of treatment he had taken fourteen treatments, and the frequency of administration was relaxed. He was now completely free of chest pain and could sleep without his sleeping pills. He had stopped the routine use of Valium, taking a pill once or twice a week if he felt it was needed.

At this time a regular daily aerobic exercise program was prescribed. At first he was monitored electronically while walking a treadmill in the clinic. He was taught how fast to walk, how to maintain the prescribed pulse level and he was encouraged to continue this routine daily.

The weather in Kansas City was still too cold for a patient with his problems to exercise outdoors. Mr. M., however, was not to be outdone. He went to a new shopping center with a heated, enclosed mall and did his walking there, early in the morning before the stores opened. It was not long before he had talked other patients into meeting there for early morning exercises. The management of the shopping center made them an official "club" and issued membership cards and coupons entitling members of the group to have breakfast at reduced prices, early movie discounts and other considerations.

Mr. M., feeling greatly improved, went back to his family physician for examination. He said he wanted him to see what EDTA had done. The doctor told him he was really no better than when he left the hospital and that the treatment was useless. The patient was very depressed when reporting this to me. I could not believe his doctor would say this, after reexamining him.

"Mr. M., go back to your doctor and ask him to repeat your treadmill electrocardiogram test," I said, "then we can get a copy of your progress for comparison. We have the hospital's initial report and we have our treadmill report when you first began treatment here. We'll see what's going on."

"I'll do it right now, Doc, if I can use your phone."

This patient went back to his doctor of twenty years, the cardiologist, at the same hospital and he had a repeat treadmill ECG performed. The patient said he could walk as fast as the machine would go at the maximum elevation it could be set and had no chest pain. After he had been walking the treadmill for thirty minutes or so, the doctor walked briskly out of the room without saying a word.

Following the standard procedure we sent an authorized request for a copy of the test information, signed by the patient. After eight weeks and several phone calls, the information had not arrived. One day Mr. M., now angry at the stalling tactics, went to the hospital and again signed a records authorization form. The results of the treadmill arrived a few

Just How Important is Chelation Therapy? 129

days later. When compared to the initial test there was an evident excellent improvement in this man's heart. The functional level of energy utilized was greatly improved. Clinically the patient was without limitation. He was now jogging four miles daily.

Psychologically however, he still had some doubt.

"After all," he told me, "they all said the same thing, and they are specialists."

"Mr. M.," I replied, "the specialists also told you that you would not live three months unless you had the bypass surgery. You do remember that, don't you?"

"Doc," he said, "I believe you, I really do. It's just that my mind is not convinced with enough certainty to relax about this thing."

"Well," I said, "If you want the certainty, and are willing to accept the expense and the risk, why don't you go back to the hospital where they did that coronary angiogram and have it repeated?"

"That's what I was thinking. I believe that's what I have to do."

This case demonstrates the tremendous psychological strain on the mind of the coronary disease patient.

Mr. M. went back to the same group of doctors who performed his initial coronary angiography, requesting a repeat test to be done. After conferring on the phone with the patient's family doctor (who referred him for the first angiogram) they refused to repeat the test stating it was too risky. The patient stated he would sign a statement absolving them and the hospital of all risk and he was willing to pay for the test. They would not perform the test.

It is my feeling they did not want radiographic proof of the improvement in their patient's coronary blood flow in their files. It would be proof, in their record files, of the efficiency of EDTA chelation therapy.

Mr. M. is in fine health today, still jogging and still working daily. He refuses to take the elevator at work, walking four flights of stairs five or six times daily as required by his job. He has referred several of his friends and his wife for treatment.

18
Chelation Can Cure

The American Academy of Medical Preventics (AAMP) teaches the chelation treatment technique to physicians. I have been honored to serve on the board of trustees of AAMP for two years. My partner, Dr. Charles J. Rudolph, Ph.D., D.O., also has served on that board.

Great progress has been made in teaching doctors the treatment. There are approximately 3,000 physicians using the procedure to the great benefit of their patients. Their greatest priority at present, as I see it, is to require their members to publish their findings in the medical literature.

The man on the street must also be made aware of this treatment and its great benefits. He can then inquire and decide if he would rather try this as an alternative to more drastic stop-gap treatment. At present, the medical establishment appears to be keeping this information from him. AAMP has only scratched the surface of progress in this area. The effort must be greatly expanded and enlarged.

Regarding physicians, the man on the firing line is the referring doctor. He is the man on the bottom of the medical ladder, the primary physician, the man who sees the patients first, the man who decides what to do for the patient. After he examines and evaluates the condition, he refers the patient on to the specialist, the surgeon or the hospital.

These two groups, primary physicians and patients, are the real power that can bring changes in this country's pitiful record of degenerative disease treatment. Pressure generated by their demands can reverse this loss of function in our people once afflicted.

EDTA chelation treatment has withstood the fires of challenge, criticism and time. It must be recognized and become as familiar as aspirin to the people if we are ever to climb out of the muck of medical mediocrity. Every patient should be offered information about the alternatives to drug therapy and surgery: EDTA chelation therapy.

In the early dawn of medicine, "physician" meant teacher. I believe this should be so today. People need to know alternative medical treatment plans, not just one "treatment of choice" blindly dispensed even though results are poor or nonexistent.

For these reasons, all physicians at our clinic routinely take the chelation story to other states, cities, towns, organizations, clubs or groups.

THE PEORIA LECTURE

During the years that I have been lecturing to physicians, paramedical groups and the public, people for the most part have been quite receptive. It is only that the occasional audience has been intimidated, threatened or otherwise influenced not to listen. Typically, it is in a small town, for this maneuver would backfire in a larger area. Once a patient from that town (who had previously been unable to win the battle against a serious chronic disease) obtains reversal of illness and regains healthy function, people are eager to listen. This is what happened in Peoria.

I was invited to Peoria, Illinois, to speak about EDTA chelation. Five weeks before my arrival, my sponsors had submitted a notice to their newspaper outlining the theory and method of treatment for cardiovascular disease. They hoped it would be printed. The newspaper did not choose to print the announcement of my talk. They said their medical advisors thought the treatment was worthless and unheard of by people of this small city.

The lecture was held at the Holiday Inn, where a small meeting room with blackboard, lectern, microphone and chairs for thirty people had been set up. People began trickling into the room forty-five minutes before I was to speak. Soon the room was filled. The manager of the motel was not concerned. He opened the accordian-like partition that separated our meeting room from a larger one. People continued to stream in. Four members of the motel staff were hard pressed to add more chairs. Soon the extra space was filled.

A third space was opened and quickly filled. Three members of my staff who had come with me, were pressed into service. They squeezed as many chairs as possible into that lecture hall. As soon as a chair was placed, it was filled.

And still they came. A doctor visiting from Florida (who had also come along on this trip), began to scavenge for more chairs now in short supply. He brought them from the lobby, from the cocktail lounge and even from other meeting rooms, if there was an unused chair.

The parking lot of the motel was jammed with cars. A nearby exit ramp of the freeway was jammed bumper to bumper with cars attempting to enter the motel parking lot. Traffic was backing up on the freeway. Two state police cars finally closed the exit ramp. A third sealed off the motel entrance. We were told that the crowd numbered more than three hundred, ten times more than expected.

The lecture ended by 9:00 p.m. Questions and answers from the audience, however, lasted until 11:30 p.m.

On balance, over the years, I have had more positive reaction than negative when speaking to the public. There is no other way to carry the story of chelation to the people. Medical conservatism will procrastinate thirty to sixty years when a new medical treatment or diagnostic approach appears. It took fifty years for the profession to recognize the worth of the electrocardiograph machine.

Theodore Roosevelt said it all: "It is not the critic who counts, not the man who points out how the strong man stumbles, or where the doer of deeds could have done them better. The credit belongs to the man who is actually in the arena, whose face is marred by dust and sweat and blood; who strives valiantly; who errs, and comes short again and again, but who does actually strive to do the deeds; who knows the great enthusiasms, the great devotions; who spends himself in a worthy cause; who, at best, knows in the end the triumph of high achievement, and who, at worst, if he fails, at least fails while daring greatly, so that his place shall never be with cold and timid souls who know neither victory nor defeat."

The aim of learning is not the mere accumulation of knowledge. The aim of learning is action. For thirty years or more, EDTA chelation treatment has been used successfully in this country. It's time all physicians make common use of it for their chronically ill patients. Of all the forces that make a better world, none is so indispensable or powerful as hope. Without hope men are only half alive. With it, they dream, think and work. It is my intent to fan the coals and embers of hope for the chronically ill. With persistence they can find their way to a physician trained by the American College of Advancement in Medicine, who can lighten or remove this burden from their lives. There is nothing more satisfying than seeing these formerly "hopeless" patients regain their strength, function and mentation.

Chelation physicians are probably the happiest in the medical profession. They are cheerful yet caring. Most admit enjoying what they are accomplishing. Is it because they are successful in the area of medicine where most physicians fail? People rarely succeed at anything unless they have fun doing it.

Alfred Adler said it nicely: "It is the individual who is not interested in his fellow men who has the greatest difficulties in life and provides the greatest injury to others. It is from among such individuals that all human failures spring."

Working at Boston University Medical Center, Dr. Deiter M. Kramsch and co-workers proved, in a paper published in *Science,* volume 213, September 1981, that calcium in artery tissue is the causative agent of atherosclerosis. They state that inhibition of the calcium flux into arterial tissue (where it can become deposited), is absolutely essential for the prevention of atherosclerosis. They further state that agents capable of regulating calcium flux and extracellular build-up in arteries may prevent atherosclerosis, even when abnormal conditions in the bloodstream, such as abnormally high cholesterol and unfavorable concentration of lipoproteins are present.

Cardiovascular disease, the leading cause of death in the United States and other industrialized nations, is a glaring example of futile, incompetent research efforts and wasted treatment dollars.

What has not been fully appreciated is that all, or nearly all, of the atherosclerosis generating processes require abundant calcium for energy to process. The lynchpin to the whole process of hardening of the arteries resulting in loss of blood circulation to vital tissue, is directing calcium to behave in its proper manner. The key to taming this scourge of civilization is an anti-calcium agent, a chelating agent. EDTA is this agent. The job can be done in spite of increased cholesterol or lipoproteins in the blood.

A great many studies have shown that diets high in cholesterol could induce atherosclerosis, but low fat diets which lowered blood cholesterol did not prevent atherosclerosis or heart disease. Something other than cholesterol must be important, and that something, the Boston investigators suggest, may be calcium. If one were to inhibit the intake of inorganic calcium, one would also inhibit the formation of atherosclerosis. My personal experience confirms this observation.

The communication barrier between researchers and practicing physicians sometimes seems insurmountable. To ignore this treatment of cardiovascular disease is unconscionable stupidity. Too many patients are being lost or sidelined unnecessarily.

In an attempt to offer practicing physicians the opportunity to see first hand the effect of EDTA chelation therapy on patients that they themselves have examined and diagnosed, the following letter was sent to the thirty-three cardiologists listed in the yellow pages of the Kansas City telephone book.

Dear Doctor:

For more than thirty years EDTA chelation therapy has been highly effective for the control and reversal of cardiovascular disease in the populations of the United States. This begins our twenty-first year of continuous experience with this treatment. Recently, we have begun a program to publish our findings of the great benefits of this synthetic amino acid treatment to patients with degenerative cardiovascular diseases.

As you know, this treatment is not taught in medical schools in the United States. This is unfortunate, because physicians are unable to learn the tremendous benefits that can be given to the cardiovascular patient. The EDTA chelation therapy program removes arterial metastic plaque calcium, safely lowers lipids more rapidly than any drug program, lowers abnormally high blood pressure, stabilizes cellular membrane chemistry, restores arterial and venous circulation, reverses gangrene, removes toxic metals such as lead, prevents platelet aggregation, smoothes arrhythmias, improves kidney function, shortens the P-R interval and reduces (or eliminates) S-T depression as seen on the treadmill ECG test. This is a partial list of benefits.

I believe you will agree that a single treatment modality that offers so many benefits to a patient deserves a serious personal investigation.

It is unfortunate, but medicine seems to suppress EDTA chelation therapy even though they have no valid scientific reason. None of its detractors have ever treated patients with EDTA.

It is our hope that we can find one doctor with foresight and open-minded flexibility who will accept a challenge to the prevailing customary and usual treatment approach to cardiovascular disease.

If you desire first hand information, we could cooperate on a study of cardiovascular patients. Our group would treat a series of your patients, examined and diagnosed by you before and after EDTA chelation therapy. These patients would be returned to your care following completion of EDTA chelation therapy.

Another group of your patients, receiving your usual treatment and completely under your care, would serve as a control group.

Should you desire to begin such a study, please call or write us without delay so that the details may be worked out and the study begun.

Sincerely,
[signed]
E.W. McDonagh, D.O.
McDonagh Medical Center, Inc.

In the eight weeks after those letters were sent, only two replies were received. The first consisted of these six words hastily scribbled across the top of our letter:

"You people are dishonest and insane."

I don't know what this learned cardiologist meant by those words. Perhaps he believed we were lying when we said EDTA was beneficial to the cardiovascular system and were crazy to use it.

The second reply came about a month later. This one page letter was written by a doctor who said he was "shocked" to learn that EDTA could do so many beneficial things. He said we should inform the Secretary of Health and Human Services, Washington, D.C.

It was a polite way to answer the letter and dodge the issue.

Do they really care? Are heart specialists really interested in an efficient method of helping their patients? This was a chance for them to participate and observe the advantage of this treatment over conventional care.

The man with experience is never at the mercy of the man with an argument, it has been said. Every cardiologist in Kansas City, however, chose to continue inadequate piecemeal symptom treatment, instead of attempting to gain additional experience in treating cardiovascular patients.

It is a sorry state of mind when one has no desire to evaluate another way to treat cardiovascular disease. I feel certain these physicians will continue to condemn EDTA chelation therapy despite the fact that not one of them has ever used it.

On the other hand, it is the patient's right to have a non-toxic, highly effective and safe treatment available at a reasonable cost. EDTA chelation therapy is that treatment.

When enough patients demand chelation it will be offered without resistance by most physicians. Until then, doctors will resist. It is to their economic advantage.

Public pressure can drag them, (kicking and screaming if necessary), into a world where the majority of chronic degenerative diseases can be prevented and reversed with greater ease and at less cost than present methods.

19
Two Miles in Winter

Success is being able to live your life in your own way. The great majority of our populace cannot do this because of degenerative disease.

Increased amounts of money have been spent yearly seeking a way out of this dilemma, yet progressively more people are slowed, sidelined or eliminated from life's mainstream. Is it because we lack the resources or knowledge to overcome these maladies? I think not.

Must civilized man accept the prediction of more heart and artery disease? Are degenerative diseases the normal consequence of our society? I believe these diseases are unnecessary, and this kind of thinking unwise.

Should we await the discovery of new miracle drugs, or a futuristic treatment approach to extract us, in the nick of time, from our predicament? The answer is *no.* A treatment process called EDTA chelation therapy has been available in this country for the past thirty years. It is more effective than any other treatment. Results are a high quality, long lasting functional improvement.

Chelation neutralizes and removes the earliest and most basic cause of degenerative disease in the human body. Safe, thorough removal of the occluding materials that stick to the inside of the arteries is accomplished all over the body. Organs that have lost function because of circulatory embarrassment have their function restored, without the use of drugs.

EDTA chelation therapy is greatly beneficial to the kidneys as we have shown in scientific, published studies. Waste products of cellular metabolism are efficiently eliminated, removing another stress factor that contributes to degenerative disease. Drugs cannot do this.

Downstream of an arterial occlusion, or narrowing, tissue cells are deprived of nutrients and oxygen normally supplied by the bloodstream. This is corrected.

The cellular membrane's ability to function normally, that is, to allow access to certain necessary materials and exclude harmful ones, is restored. Excessive inorganic calcium is removed from arteries, organs, muscles, joints and cells. The heart cells, for example, function more efficiently with less effort, as a result of EDTA chelation therapy. Profound improvement in seemingly impossible disease states is the usual treatment result.

Patients bedridden with advanced diabetic gangrene of the feet or legs are saved from the tragedy of watching the condition deteriorate until there is only one option left to prevent death: amputation. Chelation with EDTA has salvaged innumerable legs and lives. These patients return to fully functional, normal lives.

Coronary artery disease responds in a similar manner. Most patients can avoid coronary artery bypass surgery and their heart muscle cells revive and function efficiently once again. Occasionally a patient might be seen in an extremely advanced state of coronary occlusive disease and because chelation results might take weeks or months the patient might not have available, surgery is advised. The number of these cases, however, is extremely small.

New patients who have survived coronary bypass surgery will benefit greatly too. They will be able to prevent the new vessel grafts from plugging up and obtain all the other benefits to their body chemistry as well.

Another area of medical ineffectiveness is diabetes mellitus. The condition results in early, advanced occlusion in the arteries in most areas of the body. Kidney disease, impotency, blindness, resistant infections, heart attacks, strokes, gangrene and a host of other maladies are seen earlier and more frequently in these patients. Medicine has been studying the disease frantically and furiously for more than sixty years, yet no real progress has been made in prevention and treatment. Oral drugs and several kinds of insulin are available, but they merely control blood sugar. They do not reverse damage to the arteries or organs. EDTA chelation therapy on the other hand, does.

The diabetic state is a cocklebur under the saddle of medicine. Try as they may, researchers and practicing physicians have not been able to reverse insidious diabetic destruction to the cellular membranes that comprise the body's vital organs.

Now and then, medical public relations blurbs are heard or seen in the public media, ballyhooing a new synthetic insulin, or how much smoother the blood sugar can be if the patient is hooked up to an artificial insulin pump. Or, the development of a vaccine to prevent viral infection of the pancreatic islet cells and thus *prevent* certain viral induced diabetic cases from developing. This could help a few, but not the vast majority of inherited cases.

The public is led to believe that medicine is truly eliminating the disease, but in truth, it is not. Medicine concentrates on diagnostic gadgetry development and on newer ways to control diseases, because these are generators of profit and because these are perceived to be within the traditions of today's medical thinking. That thinking, of course, is why we wallow in the sorry state of epidemic chronic disease. Adhering to the maxim, "If it ain't broke, don't fix it," medicine apparently shuts its eyes as degenerative disease develops, opening them only when the patient is sufficiently sick.

But does any of this ballyhoo help doctors reverse degenerative changes in diabetic patients? Conventional conservative attempts are still being tried, but unfortunately progress is nearly nonexistent. To give credit to those persevering in research, they are working hard in the field, but they look at the problem from the wrong end of the telescope.

Surveying the medical literature of diabetes, we found six hundred papers published within the last eighteen months.

This tremendous activity confirms the fact that the medical establishment, in spite of all the prior years of research and with the renewed frenzy of current studies being published, has no answer to the problem.

Yet the answer is EDTA chelation therapy. The reversal of diabetic damage and the prevention of further deterioration by this treatment modality is truly remarkable. For more than twenty years I have witnessed the salvage and return to normal function of innumerable kidneys, eyes and legs that would have been lost with conventional treatment.

These results are not few in number. They number in the thousands. Yet, with chelation, patients can expect this result. None of these cases could be considered an exceptional case that "might have healed by itself."

Damaged hearts and brains are strengthened, revived and healed. Function once thought to be lost forever, is restored. Most important, future heart and brain infarction is prevented in most cases. The terror of gangrene is eradicated. This problem is easily solved.

Detractors of the treatment are quick to scoff at this treatment, just as they have scoffed at every new idea since the dawn of civilization. There will always be more people who get perverse satisfaction in attempting to tear down, than those who attempt to build up. This is true in every field of endeavor, and indeed, I would be concerned if there were none in the field of EDTA chelation therapy. The loudest critics are usually those most ignorant, those who have never treated a patient with EDTA.

Be careful you do not become influenced by these people. Do not allow your respect for a person's titles or credentials in one field of endeavor to color your judgment or appraisal of a treatment in which he has no expertise. Unless the critic of chelation therapy has sufficient personal experience in administering the treatment, he must be considered ignorant in his attempt to degrade it.

If your $10,000 wrist watch needs repair, would you take it to a blacksmith because he is considered the best blacksmith in the business?

Within the past year or two, other medically oriented

writers have been attempting to inform the public about the great benefits of EDTA chelation therapy. These efforts are to be encouraged. Their articles and books are an important part of the effort we must all participate in to make chelation therapy commonly available.

Most of these writers, however, cannot state the case strongly, or with sufficient credibility because they have not administered the treatment to human patients. What they say, therefore, is second hand knowledge. What I have said in this book is based on more than twenty-four years of daily chelation practice.

If a doctor is truly concerned about his patients and he honestly wants to salvage patients from the scourge of degenerative chronic disease, he must investigate EDTA chelation therapy with an open, flexible mind. When he sets aside his preconceived notions regarding the *proper* way to treat disease and allows his intellect, integrity and heart to exert valid influence on his thinking, he will not be able to deny the obvious value of the therapy.

Many patients whose disease is advanced beyond medicine's capacity to help them, can be aided synergistically by applying EDTA chelation therapy with the "treatment of choice." Greater progress can be realized in this manner than if each treatment modality is applied separately. Later, the drug therapy can be reduced gradually until it is eliminated and the patient's recovery will accelerate as a result of continuing chelation treatment.

One such patient, a very advanced diabetic man, age sixty-nine, with arthritis, gangrene of both great toes and feet, hypertensive vascular disease and generalized atherosclerosis, was also suffering from an eye condition called macular degeneration. He was legally blind and could see only ten to fifteen feet. He had suffered one previous heart attack and had chest pain radiating into the left arm intermittently. He could not walk due to the pain of gangrene. His carotid arteries were severely occluded on both sides of the neck and he was in danger of a stroke.

His surgeon wanted to amputate one leg, then three months later he planned to take the other. He did not want the patient to take chelation therapy. At the patient's request, I called the surgeon to explain the treatment.

After a lengthy conversation during which I contrasted the obvious safety of chelation compared to surgery with a general anesthetic and after citing the medical literature on chelation, he was not convinced. I went through the many papers written by our group. I explained that should chelation fail, the patient's arteries and organs would be improved significantly. Should the gangrenous leg still require amputation, the patient would be a better surgical candidate. He would survive the operation and heal well afterward.

The surgeon was unrelenting. Finally I said, "Doctor, if this was your father, wouldn't you want to give him every chance to save his legs?"

That finally did the trick. The firmness in his voice softened and he became more interested in the merits of the discussion.

We treated this patient with good results. His insulin was reduced five units per week. Originally controlled with sixtyeight units of insulin, his maintainence dosage was lowered to six units daily. He became fully functional and resumed his old business, walking with a cane. His vision improved greatly, as did his mental function.

This case demonstrates that even in the most advanced cases, normal function can be restored. And normal function is really what it's all about, isn't it?

Most people in the United States do not have normal function. They don't have the energy, or ability to work, play or love as they would like. They can't accomplish their aims and ambitions when chronic deterioration saps their energy.

Normal function allows us to pursue our goals to their conclusion. We can move about with no discomfort or worry throughout the entire day. We have no pain, stiffness, irritability, nervous tension or other pressures that we can't handle. Normal function results when the cells, organs and systems are properly nourished and able to work as designed. Feelings of fulfillment and satisfaction and enjoyment from everything life may present are commonly seen in people with normal, healthful body functions.

The reason for this book is to help others regain normal health and function when they need help beyond what is available via generally accepted medical methods.

Every mile is really two miles in winter.

For further information:

McDonagh Medical Center
2800A Kendallwood Parkway
Kansas City, MO 64119
816-453-5940

References in Alphabetical Order

1. Aldersberg, D., *Obesity, Fat Metabolism and Diabetes. Diabetes* 7:8, 236-243, May-June 1958.

2. American College of Advancement in Medicine, 6151 West Century Boulevard, Suite 1114, Los Angeles, California 90045.

3. *American Medical News,* June 17, 1974, page 18.

4. Axelrod, A., *Immune Processes in Vitamin Deficiency States, American Journal of Clinical Nutrition,* 24, 265, 1971.

5. Baker, H. Frank, S. Feingold, et al., *Vitamins, Total Cholesterol and Triglycerides in 642 New York School Children, American Journal Clinical Nutrition,* 20, 850, 1967.

6. Becker, R.R., et al., *Ascorbic Acid Deficiency and Cholesterol Synthesis, Journal American Chemical Society,* Vol. 23, pages 27-30, 1970.

7. Bland, J., Ph.D., *The Justification for Vitamin Supplementation,* Northwest Diagnostic Services, P.O. Box 6742, Bellevue, Washington 98007.

8. Blumenthal, H.T., et al., *American Journal of Pathology,* 20655, 1944.

9. Bolick, L.E., and Blankenhorn, D.H., *A Quantitative Study of Coronary Artery Calcification, American Journal Pathology,* 39:511, 1960.

10. Bolt, R.J., Tupper, C.J. and Mallery, O.T., Jr. *An Appraisal of Periodic Health Examinations, Archives Industrial Health* 12:4, 420-434, October 1955.

11. Borhani, N.O., *Screening Tests Find Longshoremen With Organized Medical Follow-up, American Journal Public Health* 42:12, 1552-1567, December 1952.

12. Brucknerova, O. and Tulacek, J., *Chelation in the Treatment of Occlusive Atherosclerosis, Unitr. Lek,* 18:7, 29, 1972.

13. Cake, M.H., Sondo, D. and Litwark, G., *Effect of Pyridoxal Phosphate on DNA Binding Site of Glucocorticoid Receptors, Journal Biological Chemistry,* 253, 4886, 1978.

14. Carroll, B.E., Kurlander, A.B. and Nester, H.G., Multiple Screening Pilot Study. *Report of Indianapolis, Indiana Project, Public Health Report* 6:12, 1180-1184, December 1956.

15. Casdorph, H.R., *EDTA Chelation Therapy Efficacy in Arteriosclerotic Heart Disease, Journal Holistic Medicine,* Volume 3:1, Spring/Summer 1981.

16. Cheraskin, E., M.D., D.M.D., Fingsdorf, W.M., Jr., D.M.D. and Clark, J.W., D.D.S., *Diet and Disease,* Keats Publishing, Inc., New Canaan, Connecticut.

17. Chidlowski, J.A. and Thunassi, J.W., *Pyridoxal Phosphate Induced Alterations in Glucocorticoid Receptor Conformation, Biochemistry,* 18, 2378, 1979.

18. Collen, M.F. and Linden, C., *Screening in a Group Practice Prepaid Medical Care Plan, Journal Chronic Diseases* 2:4, 400-408, October 1955.

19. Culbert, R.W. and Jawbziner, H., *What Does the School Physician See? American Journal Public Health* 40:5, 567-574, May 1950.

20. Entmacher, P.S. and Marks, H.H., *Diabetes in 1964, A World Survey. Diabetes* 14:4, 212-223, April 1965.

21. Elsom, K.A., Personal Communications of September 14, 1954 and February 16, 1955. Cited by Robert, N.J., *Periodic Health Maintenance Examinations.* In the *Early Detection and Prevention of Diseases in Executives,* edited by J.P. Hubbard, 1957, New York, Blakiston Division, McGraw-Hill Book Company, page 30.

22. Elsom, K.A., Sebor, S., York, T.W., Elson, I.O. and Hubbard, J.P., *Periodic Health Examination: Nature and Distribution of Newly Discovered Diseases in Executives, Journal American Medical Association* 172:1, 55-60, January 2, 1960.

23. Evans, W., *Vitamin C in Heart Failure, Lancet,* volume 1, pages 308-309, 1938.

24. Franco, S.C., *The Early Detection of Disease by Periodic Examination, Industrial Medicine and Surgery* 25:6, 251-257, June 1956.

25. Ginter, E. et al., *The Effect of Chronic Hypervitaminosis C on the Metabolism of Cholesterol and Atherogenesis in Guinea Pigs. Journal of Arteriosclerosis Research,* volume 10, pages 341-352, 1969.

26. Halstead, B.W., M.D., *The Scientific Basis of Chelation Therapy,* Golden Quill Publishers, Inc., Box 1278, Colton, California 93324.

27. Harper, H.W., M.D. and Culbert, M.L., *How You Can Beat the Killer Disease,* Arlington House, New Rochelle, New York, 1977.

28. *Heart Facts 1982,* American Heart Association, National Center, 7320 Greenville Avenue, Dallas, Texas 75231.

29. Horn, L.R., Machlin, L.J., Banker, M.O. and Brin, M., *Drug Metabolism and Vitamin Undernutriture, Archives Biophysics,* 172, 270, 1978.

30. Huth, E., Meidt, C., Vernon W., Spoondt, S. and Dohan, F.C., *Periodic Health Status Examination Program,* unpublished report, June 29, 1954. Cited by Roberts, N.J., *Periodic Health—Maintenance Examinations in the Early Detection and Prevention of Disease,* edited by J.P. Hubbard, 1957, New York, Blakiston Division, McGraw-Hill Book Company, page 30.

31. International Academy of Preventive Medicine, 34 Corporate Woods, Suite 469, 10950 Grandview, Overland Park, Kansas 66210.

32. Kurliandehekov, U.N., *Treatment of Patients with Coronary Arteriosclerosis with Unithol on Combination Decamevi, Vracg. Delo.,* 6:8, 1973.

33. Kitchell, J.R., Meltzer, L.E. and Seven, M.J., *Potential Uses of Chelation Methods in the Treatment of Vascular Diseases, Progressive Cardiovascular Disease* 3:338, 1961.

34. Klenner, F.R., (1), *The Treatment of Poliomyelitis and Other Virus Diseases with Vitamin C, Southern Medicine and Surgery,* volume 3, pages 209-214, 1949. *Massive Doses of Vitamin C and the Virus Diseases,* ibid., volume 113, pages 101-107, 1951. *The Vitamins and Massage Treatment for Acute Poliomyelitis,* ibid., volume 114, pages 194-197, 1952. *The Use of Vitamin C as an Antibiotic, Journal of Applied Nutrition,* volume 6, pages 274-278, 1953. *The Folly in the Continued Use of a Killed Polio Virus Vaccine, Tri-State Medical Journal,* pages 1-8, 1959.

35. Klenner, F.R., (2), *Virus Pneumonia and its Treatment with Vitamin C, Southern Medicine and Surgery,* volume 110, pages 36-46, 1948.

36. Krehl, W.A., *The Evaluation of Nutritional Status, Medical Clinics of North America* 48:5, 1129-1140, September 1964.

37. Lamar, C.P., *Calcium Chelation and Atherosclerosis—Nine Years Clinical Experience,* Fourteenth Annual Meeting of American College Angiology, 1968.

38. Levin, M.E. and Recant, L., *Diabetes and the Environment, Archives Environmental Health* 12:5, 621-630, May 1966.

39. Lisa, P.J., *The Great Medical Monopoly Wars,* Internatinal Institute of Natural Health Sciences, Inc., P.O. Box 5550, Huntington Beach, California 92615, 1987.

40. Lonsdale, D. and Shamberger, R., *Red Cell Transketolase As An Indication of Nutritional Deficiency, American Journal of Clinical Nutrition,* 33, 205, 1980.

41. McDonagh, E.W., Rudolph, C.J. and Cheraskin, E., *Serum Cholesterol and the Aging Process, Medical Hypotheses,* volume VII, pages 685-694, 1981.

42. McDonagh, E.W., Rudolph, C.J. and Cheraskin, E., (1), *The Effect of Intravenous Disodium EDTA Acid Upon Blood Cholesterol in a Private Practice Environment,* Journal International Academy of Preventive Medicine, volume VII, number 1, April 1982.

43. McDonagh, E.W., Rudolph, C.J. and Cheraskin, E., (2), *The Effect of EDTA Salts Plus Supportive Multi-vitamin-Trace Mineral Supplementation upon Renal Function: A Study in Serum Creatinine, Journal Holistic Medicine,* 1982.

44. McDonagh, E.W., Rudolph, C.J. and Cheraskin, E., (3), *The Homeostatic Effect of EDTA with Supportive Multivitamin-Trace Mineral Supplementation Upon High Density Lipoproteins (HDL),* Journal Osteopathic Physicians and Surgeons of California, 8:2, Spring Issue, 1982.

45. McDonagh, E.W., Rudolph, C.J. and Cheraskin, E., (4), *An Occulocerebrovasculometric Analysis of the Effect of EDTA Chelation Upon Vascular Stenosis, Journal Holistic Medicine,* May, 1982.

46. McDonagh, E.W., (5), *Hyperbaric Oxygen Therapy,* McDonagh Medical Center, 2800-A Kendall Parkway, Kansas City, Missouri 64119, 1982.

47. McDonagh, E.W., Rudolph, C.J. and Cheraskin, E., *The Influence of EDTA Salts Plus Multivitamin-Trace Mineral Therapy Upon Total Serum Cholesterol/High Density Lipoprotein Cholesterol,* Medical Hypothesis, 1983.

48. McDonagh, E.W., Rudolph, C.J., Cheraskin, E. and Wussow, D., *EDTA Chelation and Electrocardiography, Journal Holistic Medicine,* in press.

49. McDonagh Medical Center, Inc., 2800-A Kendallwood Parkway, Kansas City, Missouri 64119.

50. Moriyama, I.M., *The Change in Mortality Trends in the United States,* National Center for Health Statistics, United States Department of Health, Education and Welfare, Public Health Service Publication 1,000, Series 3:1, March 1964.

51. Muller, S.A., Brunsting, L.A. and Winlemann, R.K., *The Treatment of Scleroderma with the New Chelating Agent, Edathamil,* American Medical Association Archive Dermatology: 80, 187, 1959.

52. National Center for Health Statistics, (1), *Bed Disability Among the Chronically Limited,* United States July 1957, June 1961, Series 10:12, September 1964, Washington, D.C., Superintendent of Documents, United States Government Printing Office.

53. National Center for Health Statistics, (2), *Chronic Conditions and Activity Limitations, United States July 1961-June 1963,* Series 10:17, May 1965. Washington, D.C., Superintendent of Documents United States Government Printing Office.

54. Northwest Academy of Preventive Medicine, 15615 Bellevue, Redmond Road, Suite E, Bellevue, Washington 98008.

55. Prinz, W., Bontz, R., Bregin, B. and Hersch, M., *Effect of Ascorbic Acid Supplementation of Some Parameters of Human Immunological Defense System, Journal Vitamin Nutrition Research,* 47, 248, 1977.

56. *Reversing Degeneration and Aging Through Chelation,* McDonagh Medical Center, 2800-A Kendallwood Parkway, Kansas City, Missouri 64119, 1982 (revised).

57. Roberts, N.J., *Periodic Health-Maintainence Examination in the Early Detection and Prevention of Disease,* edited by J.P. Hubbard, 1957, New York, Blakiston Division, McGraw-Hill Book Company, pages 27-57.

58. Rudolph, C.J., *Trace Element Patterning in Degenerative Diseases, Journal International Academy Preventive Medicine,* July 1977.

59. Rudolph, C.J. and Cordas, S., *Insight Preventive Medicine: Chromium, Osteopathic Medicine,* January 1978, 3 (1), 52-57.

60. Schweiker, R.S., *Chemoprevention Now National Goal, Medical Tribune,* volume 23:13, June 30, 1982.

61. Sebrov, K.R., *Prophylaxis and Treatment of Arteriosclerosis with Ascorbic Acid, Terapevitcheskii Arkhiv* (Moskva), volume 28, pages 58-65, 1956.

62. Selye, Q., *Calciphylaxis,* Chicago, Illinois, University of Chicago Press, 1960.

63. Shaffer, C.F., *The Diuretic Effect of Ascorbic Acid, Journal American Medical Association,* volume 124, pages 700-701, 1944.

Ascorbic Acid as a Diuretic, Lancet, volume 2, page 186, 1944.

Shaffer, C.F., et al., *The Use of Oral Mercuhydrin Combined Ascorbic Acid in Cardiac Decompensation, American Journal Medical Sciences,* volume 219, pages 674-678, 1950.

64. Sheps, C.G., *The Dynamics of Medical Care,* 1960, Evanston, Illinois, Association of American Medical Colleges.

65. Spies, T.D., *Some Recent Advances in Nutrition, Journal American Medical Association* 167:6, 675-690, June 7, 1958.

66. Stewart, W.H., *Who Gets What Care and How?* In the *Health Care Issue* of the 1960, 1963, Group Health Insurance, Inc., 221 Park Avenue South, New York, New York.

67. Stone, I., *The Healing Factor, "Vitamin C" Against Disease,* Grosset and Dunlop, New York, 1982.

68. *The Arizona Republic, Joint Panel Agrees to Cut Deduction for Medical Costs,* Saturday, August 14, 1982, Phoenix, Arizona.

69. The President's Commission of Heart Disease, Cancer and Stroke, *Report to the President; A National Program to Conquer Heart Disease, Cancer and Stroke,* volume 1, December 1964, Washington, D.C., Superintendent of Documents, United States Government Printing Office.

70. *The Wall Street Journal,* Tuesday, July 27, 1982, page 25.

71. Thompson, C.E. and Staack, H.F., *Executive Health-Diagnostic Study of 600 Executives, Industrial Medicine and Surgery* 25:4, 175-176, April 1956.

72. United States Department of Health, Education and Welfare, (1), *Health, Education and Welfare Trends,* 1963, Washington, D.C., Superintendent of Documents United States Government Printing Office.

73. United States Department of Health, Education and Welfare, (2), *Public Health Service Health Statistics from United States National Health Survey, Selected Dental Findings in Adults by Age, Race and Sex, United States, 1960-1962,* Series 11:7, February 1965, Washington, D.C., Superintendent of Documents United States Government Printing Office.

74. Wade, L., *Physical Examinations for Executives, Archives Industrial Health* 17:3, 175-179, March 1958.

75. Walker, M., *Chelation Therapy,* M. Evans and Company, New York, New York 10017, 1980.

76. Weinerman, E.R., Breslow, L., Belloc, N.B., Waybur, A. and Milmore, B.K., *Multiphasic Screening of Longshoremen with Organized Medical Follow-up, American Journal Public Health* 42:12, 1552-1567, December 1952.

77. Willis, G.C. and Fishman, S., *Ascorbic Acid Content of Human Arterial Tissue, Canadian Medical Association Journal,* volume 72, pages 500-503, 1955.

78. Young, W.O., *Dental Health in Hollinshead, The Survey of Dentistry,* 1961, Washington, D.C., American Council on Education, pages 5-16.

INDEX

M

Magnesium, chelate of, 10
McDonagh Medical Center, 28, 29, 31, 32, 49, 61, 89, 107, 113, 121, 127, 137
McDonagh, E.W., 31, 32, 137
Medical Costs and the Drug Industry, 20
Medical insurance, 24
Medical philosophy, 5
Medical Tribune, 67, 101
Medical World News, 12
Medicine, modern, deficits of, 22-32
Meltzer, L.E., 12
Metastatic calcium deposits, 9, 13
Midwest Health and Lifestyle, 107
Millman, Marsha, 5
Minnesota Mining and Manufacturing, 6
Missouri Association of Osteopathic Physicians and Surgeons, 29, 30
Modern Concepts of Cardiovascular Disease, 45
Moriyama, Iwao M., 44
Muller, S.A., 12
Multiple sclerosis, 113
Myocardial infarction, 5

N

National Academy of Sciences, 99
National Cancer Institute, 101
National Institute of Mental Health, 68
Nephrocalcinosis, 9
Neuroenzymes, 55
Neurohormones, 55
New England Journal of Medicine, 2, 84, 113, 121
Nicotine, 6
Northwestern Medical School, 99
Nutrition Research Laboratories, 83

O

Obesity, 6
Occlusion, 47
Occulocerebrovasculometric Analysis of the Effect of EDTA Chelation Upon Vascular Stenosis, 107
Occulocerebrovasculometry, 45
Office of Health Statistics Analysis, 44
Ohio State University, 57

P

Palliation, drug, 5
Paralysis, 64

Pauling, Linus, 101
People, 99
Peoria lecture, 132
Peripheral vascular disease, symptoms of, 72
Philosophy, medical, 5
Physiotherapy, 59
Plethysmography, 45
Prophyrias, 9
Prostatic calcinosis, 9
Providence Hospital (Detroit), 11
Public Health Service, 44
Pulmonary embolism, 39

Q

Questionnaire, clinic, 114-119

R

Radiation, 8
Reversing Degeneration and Aging Through Chelation, 91
Rudolph, Charles Jr., 29, 30, 73, 104, 127, 131

S

Salt, 6
Saphenous vein, 6
Schuller, Robert, 96
Schwartz, Harry, 20
Schweiker, Richard S., 100
Science, 134
Scientific Basis of Chelation Therapy, The, 10
Scleroderma, 9
Selenium, 38, 39
Senility, 66-71
Seven, M.J., 12
Shortness of breath, 5
Sinoatrial block, 49
Sinus bradycardia, 49
Sinus tachycardia, 49
Smoking, (see tobacco)
Social Security, 24, 71
Sokoloff, Louis, 67, 68
Spies, T.D., 99
Stewart, William H., 44
Stone, Irwin, 90
Stress test, 105-106
Stroke, 51-65, risk factors, 57, risk-prone patient, 57
Sugar, 6
Surgeon general, 26
Symptoms, treatment of, 5